Trauma-Informed Parenting Program

Trauma-Informed Parenting Program

TIP^s for Clinicians to Train Parents of Children Impacted by Trauma & Adversity

Carryl P. Navalta

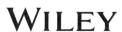

This edition first published 2022
© 2022 John Wiley & Sons, Inc.

The right of Carryl P. Navalta to be identified as the author of this work has been asserted in accordance with law.

Registered Office
John Wiley & Sons, Inc., 111 River Street, Hoboken, NJ 07030, USA

Editorial Office
111 River Street, Hoboken, NJ 07030, USA

For details of our global editorial offices, customer services, and more information about Wiley products visit us at www.wiley.com.

Wiley also publishes its books in a variety of electronic formats and by print-on-demand. Some content that appears in standard print versions of this book may not be available in other formats.

Library of Congress Cataloging-in-Publication Data applied for

Paperback ISBN: 9781119772361

Cover Design: Wiley
Cover Image: © seamind224/Shutterstock

Set in 10/12pt and WarnockPro by Straive, Chennai, India

I am deeply honored to dedicate this book to my late father, Feliciano S. Navalta, Jr., M.D. The love and support he provided to his family, friends, colleagues, and patients were unparalleled.
I love you, Dad!

Contents

Foreword

Over the last 25 years, I have worked as a clinical researcher interested largely in the areas of treatment development, implementation, and dissemination. In doing this work, I have seen first-hand how important it is to train and support the clinical workforce, particularly community providers. Remarkably, I met Dr. Carryl P. Navalta nearly 10 years ago as part of a national initiative designed to improve access to and quality of care for youth who have experienced trauma, the National Child Traumatic Stress Network. We were actually working on a study that compared child-perpetrator relationships for physical and sexual abuse and disparate mental health outcomes. Dr. Navalta has continued on his journey to explore how trauma, abuse, and other adversities create a heavy weight for families to carry and how care-giving relationships play an important role in the youth's response.

Whether you are a seasoned clinician or someone just getting started with their clinical career, it is important to understand how trauma affects children, adolescents, and their families. Specifically, clinicians need to be able to address the rippling effects that trauma and adversity have on the developing brains and behaviors of children and adolescents. This book on the *Trauma-Informed Parenting Program* is a valuable resource that guides clinicians on how to empower parents in their role as caregivers, enhance their child's response, and develop emotion regulation skills. The book summarizes key research findings and contextualizes this information with relevant history and background information while answering common questions from beginning to end. It also uses easy to understand language and provides the reader with a roadmap with helpful tips and strategies to use along the way. Of course, as a self-proclaimed foodie, my favorite parts are the delicious recipes for success – something we can all use in doing this challenging but rewarding work.

Chapters 3 and 4 are undoubtedly the bread and butter of the book. They address two critical concepts (case conceptualization and treatment planning) that are the basis for effective treatments and interventions. Far too often, when clinicians skip these critical steps of assessment and case formulation they do not obtain the clinical understanding needed to guide treatment selection and implementation. Failure to understand the primary problem and their context can lead to the wrong selection of treatments and can be potentially harmful to the child and family. The treatment planning section really addresses how clinicians can individualize treatment for that specific child/family based on the assessment information gathered. This approach goes beyond a "cookie cutter" approach to tailor interventions to address specific problems as well as cultural and developmental considerations related to their trauma exposure and specific response. Understanding these two concepts alone is worth the price of the book.

As the pandemic continues to unfold and the mental health crisis for youth worsens, we need resources such as this book in our back pockets. I wish I had this easy read back in the day when I was learning how to effectively treat the children, adolescents and families who trusted me with their clinical care. Perhaps now more than ever, we need practical guides and resources to assist our workforce as many are struggling to respond to the increased demand that is a result of the mounting mental health crisis for our youth. Likewise, as the syndemics of COVID-19, racial injustice, and violence and trauma continue to plague our nation, we need resources with tips and strategies that complement existing treatment manuals aimed at parent training, screening and assessment, and intervention delivery that address the growing complexity of the clinical cases flooding our doorsteps. Dr. Navalta's book has the potential to assist clinicians in their quest to help youth and their families live meaningful lives that are free of trauma-related symptoms and distress.

Ernestine Briggs-King, Ph.D.
Associate Professor in Psychiatry and Behavioral Sciences
Duke University School of Medicine

Acknowledgements

The work that I've done in the field of developmental adversity has been influenced by notable individuals who've shared their collective wisdoms with me. First, the late Donald J. Levis, Ph.D. emboldened me while I was a doctoral student to account for experiences of child abuse and neglect in the histories of everyone I treat as he was fiercely adamant that such maltreatment is a predominant risk factor for most (if not all) forms of psychopathology. Second, both Martin H. Teicher, M.D., Ph.D. and Glenn Saxe, M.D. underscored to me the need for clinical sensitivity and sophistication across neurobiological and social environmental contexts, respectively, to better understand and help youth impacted by exposure to trauma and adversity. Third, Bessel van der Kolk, M.D. reinforced for me the notion that we need to take a wholistic perspective with every individual we encounter but also to keep in front of our brains the reality that trauma and adversity in all forms affect society as a whole. Lastly, Susan L. Andersen, Ph.D. taught (and continues to inform) me that intervening as early in development as possible must be the overarching goal so that the youth can have the maximal chances and time to live fulfilling and meaningful lives.

About the Companion Website

This book is accompanied by a companion website:

www.wiley.com/go/navalta/tipsforclinicians

This website includes editable and downloadable versions of the forms found in this book.

1

Introduction and Foundations

At the end of this chapter, you will be able to:

- Describe the historical roots of trauma
- State how prevalent childhood trauma exposure is
- Summarize the effects of adverse childhood experiences (ACEs) on child development
- Describe dysregulation of emotions and related behaviors
- Outline the effects of ACEs on the family
- Recite the overall premise of TIP^s
- Characterize effective emotion regulation as an index of resilience

Introduction

This book was initially proposed to focus on children who've been affected by trauma on mostly an individual level, such as exposure to child abuse or neglect or other forms of interpersonal violence. However, the coronavirus/COVID-19 pandemic and its consequences have ultimately impacted, either directly or indirectly, perhaps every child on Planet Earth in what is known as mass or collective trauma. This backdrop of trauma on a global scale makes this book both timely and relevant. Perhaps at no other time in history have parents needed to be supported and guided by behavioral healthcare professionals to effectively care for and nurture their children, especially if they are experiencing negative consequences of the pandemic or other types of trauma (Putnam et al., 2015). Although long overdue, this manual is in many ways "just what the doctor ordered"!

Although the term, "trauma", is generally used to refer to a significant adverse event, how an individual child has experienced the pandemic has varied, including conditions that meet formal definitions of trauma (e.g., death of a family member) as well as situations that fall short of such definitions but

Trauma-Informed Parenting Program: TIP^s for Clinicians to Train Parents of Children Impacted by Trauma & Adversity, First Edition. Carryl P. Navalta.
© 2022 John Wiley & Sons, Inc. Published 2022 by John Wiley & Sons, Inc.
Companion Website: www.wiley.com/go/navalta/tipsforclinicians

Table 1.1 Terminology used to label exposure to trauma and adversity during childhood and adolescence[a].

Term
ACEs
Child traumatic stress
Complex PTSD
Acute vs. chronic trauma
Developmental trauma disorder
Allostatic load
Complex trauma
Chronic stress
Post-traumatic stress disorder
Toxic stress
Poly-victimization
Developmental adversity

a) Adapted from Childhood Adversity Narratives (Putnam et al., 2015).

are nevertheless highly stressful (e.g., parental job loss and resulting financial strain). This variation highlights the need to visit the historical roots of trauma before providing a contemporary account of what is now known as *adverse childhood experiences (ACEs)* or *developmental adversity* (see Table 1.1 for other similar terms).

Trauma in Historical Context

As with most behavioral health-related phenomena, the concept of trauma was first associated with adults rather than children. For example, the advent of the train and railway system during the late 1800s resulted in anxiety of the technology and the identification of new health disorders tied to railroad crashes, collisions, or other mishaps, such as *railway spine* (Trimble, 1981). In his seminal book, *On Railway and Other Injuries of the Nervous System*, Erichsen (1866) documented symptoms of injured train passengers, which today would be recognized as post-traumatic stress symptoms. Although the prevailing view was that such symptoms were caused by organic factors (e.g., Eulenberg, 1878), a few forward-thinking individuals speculated psychological reasons for them (e.g., Page, 1883).

Work in the early 1900s helped to validate the concept of trauma in adults. Hesnard (1914), for example, provided some of the earliest descriptions of post-traumatic stress symptoms in first responders when he investigated the effects of French ship explosions. These investigations were a precursor to the identification of *shell shock* in World War I military veterans. Although initially believed to be organic brain damage due to shock waves from explosions, the condition came to be ultimately understood as psychological in origin, hence the term becoming disfavored (Myers, 1915, 1940).

Influential people pre-, peri-, and post-World War II continued to shape the present understanding of trauma. Studies of World War I veterans illustrated the post-traumatic stress symptoms of those individuals exposed to combat, including physiological hyperarousal (labeled as *physioneurosis* by Kardiner, 1941). *Combat exhaustion* (i.e., psychosomatic reactions + fatigue) was identified in many World War II combat-exposed military personnel (Grinker & Spiegel, 1945), whereas *concentration camp syndrome* was observed by Hermann and Thygesen (1954) in former prisoners of war. Similarly, *war sailor syndrome* was defined in Allied Merchant Navy personnel (Askevold, 1976), who weren't physical trauma survivors but nonetheless experienced behavioral health symptoms, anxiety in particular (Hartvig, 1977).

In the 1970s, a number of syndromes associated with varied trauma exposures were examined, such as *rape trauma syndrome, Vietnam War syndrome, battered woman syndrome*, and *abused child syndrome* (Burgess & Holmstrom, 1974; Figley, 1978; Terr, 1979). In Scandinavia, studies of disasters uncovered five pathogenic factors: (a) physical injury; (b) severe danger; (c) profoundly negative experiences of witness survivors; (d) loss of close ones; and (e) responsibility trauma (Weisaeth, 1984). Although the new focus on children led to the acknowledgment of taking a developmental approach to the consequences of trauma (Terr, 1979), this emphasis was, in fact, *r*enewed in that the earlier theorizing and writings of Freud targeted the hypothesized causal role that child sexual abuse plays in the development of behavioral health problems (Freud, 1959).

Trauma and Children: The Case of Child Abuse and Neglect

Child abuse and neglect have their historical underpinnings as far back as the first century ACE. For example, Lynch (1985) referred to writings during this period suggesting that "those caring for young children were capable of physical abuse, rejection, and neglect" (p. 7). In 1962, Kempe (1962) published what is highly regarded as the initial seminal article that jump-started the clinical and scientific field of child abuse and neglect. Dr. Kempe coined the term, *battered-child syndrome*, to describe the clinical condition in which children had been physically abused, typically by a primary caregiver. He was also among the first to use the term, *trauma*, to characterize the phenomenon and recognize its role as a significant cause of childhood disability. Today, not only does this field include physical and sexual abuse, experiences of neglect and emotional abuse also fall under this generic category (related terms include *emotional maltreatment, psychological abuse,* and *psychological battering*; Navalta et al., 2008a). As a whole, child abuse and neglect are common worldwide and are the primary problems that child protective/social services address (Djeddah et al., 2000; Jud et al., 2012).

Generally speaking, trauma refers to events or experiences that involve the possibility of or actual severe physical injury or life threat. These factors that characterize trauma are highlighted in the definition of trauma found in the Diagnostic and Statistical Manual of Mental Disorders, 5th Edition (DSM-5; American Psychiatric Association, 2013a). According to the definition, trauma is exposure to *death, threatened death, actual or threatened serious injury, or actual or threatened sexual violence.* However, this narrow focus on death, injury, or violence has been expanded both in clinical practice and research (especially with children) to include experiences that do not meet formal definitions of trauma (e.g., DSM-5), but are nevertheless quite stressful (in other words, *sub-threshold* traumatic experiences). In clinical circles, the term, *little Ts,* is sometimes used by practitioners to reference such experiences (as opposed to *big Ts*).

The Advent of "Adverse Childhood Experiences"

In the mid-1990s, researchers at the United States Centers for Disease Control and Prevention (CDC) collaborated with staff from a large health maintenance organization in the state of California, Kaiser Permanente, to initiate what is presently regarded as a landmark research project on identifying key social determinants of health (and health problems) during childhood and adolescence (Felitti et al., 1998). Specifically, the investigators focused on serious adversity and how such experiences influence functioning later in life. A questionnaire was devised to assess for exposure to various adversities, including abuse, witnessing domestic violence, and serious household dysfunction. Besides assessing for a wide range of abusive and neglectful experiences, the scale also included several sub-threshold traumatic experiences (for example, parental marital discord, living with a household member who had a substance use, behavioral health, or criminal problem). Due to this combination of experiences, the investigators created the term, *adverse childhood experiences* (or *ACEs*), to encapsulate both and consequently named their study the *Adverse Childhood Experiences (ACE) Study.*

Prevalence of ACEs

ACEs know no geographical boundaries and are thus a worldwide phenomenon. Unfortunately, the extent of exposure to ACEs (especially interpersonal ones) is both appalling and unacceptable, which will continue to fuel prevention efforts to decrease their incidence, frequency, and magnitude. In the United States, state and national data are collected on the prevalence of child abuse and neglect. For example, the Children's Bureau (Administration for Children & Families, US Department of Health & Human Services) has an annual *Child Maltreatment* report that comprises data provided by each state to the National Child Abuse and Neglect Data Systems. For 2018, approximately 678,000 children were identified as abuse and neglect survivors with a prevalence rate of 9.2 per 1,000 children (9.6 per 1,000 for females; 8.7 per 1,000 for males; US Department of Health & Human Services, Administration for Children and Families, & Administration on Children, Youth, and Families, Children's Bureau, 2020). Racial and ethnic inequities were observed, with American Indian or Alaska Native children having the highest rate at 15.2 per 1,000 and African American children with the second-highest rate (14.0 per 1,000 children).

The National Incidence Study (NIS) is a congressionally mandated, periodic research effort to assess the incidence of child abuse and neglect in the United States. In collaboration with the Children's Bureau, the Office of Planning, Research, and Evaluation conducted the Fourth National Incidence Study of Child Abuse and Neglect (NIS-4; 2010)—the data for which was collected in 2005 and 2006. In contrast to the Children's Bureau annual *Child Maltreatment* report that is based on state-level data on official reports of child maltreatment, the NIS studies include cases that both are and aren't reported to the authorities to more broadly determine the incidence of child maltreatment in the United States. Using a strict definition of maltreatment (that is, demonstrable harm is present), 1 in 58 children in the United States was a survivor of maltreatment (an estimated 1,256,600 children). This finding corresponds to 17.2 per 1,000 children, which is almost twice the prevalence documented in *Child Maltreatment* (2018) but a 32% decline in the rate compared to NIS–3 (1993). Most children were exposed to neglect (61%), whereas 44% were abuse survivors (Footnote: Because the NIS classifies children in every category that applies, the sum of the components is more than 100%).

Using a more inclusive definition of maltreatment (that is, *"endangered"* children who were not yet harmed; adding children abused and neglected by non-parent adult caregivers in certain maltreatment categories as well as teenage caregivers as perpetrators of sexual abuse) resulted in markedly higher rates. Specifically, 1 in every 25 children was a maltreatment survivor, which corresponds to a rate of 40 per 1,000 children. Across types, more than three-fourths (77%; ~2,251,600 children) were neglected and 29% (~835,000 children) were abused. Within the overall neglect category, rates were in the following order: physical neglect (53%), emotional neglect (52%), and educational neglect (16%). Of the abuse survivors, 57% were physically abused, 36% were emotionally abused, and 22% were sexually abused. In nearly all cases (that is, overall maltreatment, overall abuse, overall neglect, and physical abuse), maltreatment rates for African-American children were significantly higher than for White and Latin-American children regardless of definitional standard, which is similar to the *Child Maltreatment* findings.

Of course, ACEs comprise other adversities besides child maltreatment. Since the original *ACE Study*, the list of ACEs has been expanded to ten items. Besides five types of abuse and neglect (that is, physical abuse, psychological abuse, sexual abuse, physical neglect, and emotional neglect), five other items are focused on parent- or family-related problems: parental loss through divorce, death or abandonment, parental imprisonment, parental mental health problems, parental substance use problems, and violence against the mother. Using data collected by the National Child Traumatic Stress Network (NCTSN), Pynoos et al. (2014) documented that the original ACEs were the most prevalent adversities in their sample of children and adolescents (that is, traumatic loss/bereavement/separation, domestic violence, impaired caregiver, emotional abuse, neglect, physical abuse, and sexual abuse). However, our discussions and understanding need to include other relevant adversities because they can also have negative, long-term developmental effects (Finkelhor et al., 2015a). Such ACEs comprise childhood bullying and peer victimization, isolation and peer rejection, poverty and deprivation, and exposure to community violence. Thus, the prevalence of these experiences needs to be part of our present conversation.

The second National Survey of Children's Exposure to Violence was conducted in 2011 as a follow-up to the original study. The research included a nationwide representative sample of 4,503 children and their caregivers regarding the children's exposure to violence, crime, and abuse across several major categories: conventional crime, child maltreatment, victimization by peers and siblings, sexual victimization, witnessing and indirect victimization (including exposure to community violence, family violence, and school violence and threats), and Internet victimization (Finkelhor et al., 2015b). Overall, approximately three in five children (57.7%) experienced at least one exposure to five categories of violence in the past year (physical assault, sexual victimization, maltreatment, property victimization, and witnessed or indirect violence). Table 1.2 illustrates the major findings across exposure types. Multiple exposures to violence among children and youth were documented (also known as complex trauma and poly-victimization). Specifically, almost one-half (48.4%) of the participants reported more than one type of direct or witnessed victimization in the past year—about 1 in 6 (15.1%) reported six or more types of direct or witnessed victimization, and 1 in 20 (4.9%) reported ten or more types of direct or witnessed victimization. Exposure to one type of violence, crime, or abuse increased the chance that a child had exposure to other types. In general, the risk for an additional type of exposure was increased

Table 1.2 Exposure to surveyed categories of violence.

Exposure type	Past year (%)	Lifetime (%)
Any physical assault	41.2	54.5
Any sexual victimization	5.6	9.5
Any child maltreatment	13.8	25.6
Any property victimization	24.1	40.2
Witnessing violence	22.4	39.2
Indirect exposure to violence	3.4	10.1

two- or three-fold for a past-year exposure and somewhat more for lifetime exposure.

Unique characteristics of perpetrators and survivor gender were observed. In regard to physical assaults, siblings and non-sibling peers were both common perpetrators. Assaults by siblings occurred the most among 6- to 9-year-old children (28.0% in the past year), whereas assaults by non-sibling peers were most common among 10- to 13-year-olds (23.5% in the past year), although such assaults were typical throughout childhood and adolescence. Although boys experienced more assaults overall (45.2% vs. 37.1% for girls), girls were survivors of more dating violence (4.7% vs. 1.9%).

Rates of bullying were also surveyed (the terms, *physical intimidation* and *relational aggression,* were used in the study). Within the past year, 13.7% of children and youth were physically intimidated, and 36.5% were survivors of relational aggression. Past-year rates of exposure to relational aggression and Internet/cell phone harassment were higher for girls (41.4% vs. 31.9% and 8.3% vs. 3.8%, respectively). Rates of physical intimidation in the past year differed by age, with the highest rate experienced by children younger than ten years old, although such rates for boys and girls were comparable overall. Among other victimization types occurring in the past year, relational aggression was highest for children 6-9 years old; Internet/cell phone harassment was highest for 14- to 17-year-old youth.

About one-quarter of the sample were survivors of property victimization (that is, robbery, vandalism, and theft by non-siblings; 24.1%) or had witnessed violence in the past year (22.4%), either in the family or community. More than one in five children surveyed (20.8%) witnessed a family assault over their lifetimes, with the oldest youth (ages 14-17 years) witnessing any family assault at 34.5% (28.3% witnessing one parent assaulting another). Few significant gender or age differences were seen in witnessing family assaults. The rate of witnessing a community assault for all children and youth was 16.9% in the past year and 58.9% over the lifetime of the oldest youth.

Exposure Across Development

Besides understanding the variety of ACEs that occur and their prevalence rates, the timeframe of exposure to such adversity is important to know because of the differential impact on a child's biopsychosocial development. The developmental timing of exposure to ACEs is illustrated by findings of the Developmental Victimization Survey (Finkelhor et al., 2009), which was a national telephone survey of the victimization experiences of 2,030 children and adolescents who were 2-17 years old. Overall, the mean number of victimizations during a single year increased with age, as did the percentage of children with poly-victimizations (four or more different kinds of victimization). Specifically, the mean number of different kinds of victimizations increased from about 1.7 for 2- to 5-year-olds to 3.4 for 14- to 17-year-old youth (boys experienced more kinds of victimizations than girls in the 6–9 and 10–13 age groups); the increase in polyvictimization was greatest for boys older than 6–9 years and girls older than 10–13 years.

However, some specific types of victimization were highest before adolescence and then declined. For example, assaults by siblings peaked at ages six to nine years for both boys and girls, then declined thereafter. Similarly, physical bullying was at its highest for children six to nine years old, especially for boys, and the extent of emotional bullying dropped for both boys and girls in the 14- to 17-year-old age range. In contrast, sexual victimization increased with age, especially with girls 14-17 years old.

Developmental patterns of other victimization types varied by gender. Child maltreatment also had a pattern that varied significantly by gender. Compared to girls, boys experienced more maltreatment (physical abuse, neglect, and emotional abuse) up to 13 years old. The maltreatment of girls aged 14-17 years old, however, increased significantly to a rate higher than the rate for boys. Likewise, property crime victimization of girls increased for 14- to 17-year-olds.

The results of the Developmental Victimization Survey indicate that the overall extent of victimization is high across childhood and adolescence. Although the general pattern is that victimization increases as children get older, the pattern varies depending on the specific types of victimization as well as gender (Finkelhor et al., 2009). A recent replication study validated and extended these findings by showing that increasingly complex patterns of developmental adversity occur in middle childhood and adolescence compared to early childhood (Grasso et al., 2016).

In the case of exposure to ACEs, children are not unfortunately created equal. In other words, some children are at greater risk of experiencing ACEs compared to others. Thus, we need to know as best we can who these children are so that we can intervene as early as possible to lessen the negative consequences of such adversity or, better yet, decrease the chances that ACEs actually occur.

Table 1.3 Risk factors for experiencing developmental adversity.

Factor	Descriptor
Sex	Girls are sexually abused more often than boys
Age	Older age across most abuse and neglect categories
Disability status	Children with confirmed disabilities have lower rates of physical abuse but higher rates of emotional neglect
School enrollment	Children not enrolled in school are sexually abused more often than enrolled children
Parental job status	Unemployment
Family financial status	Low socioeconomic status
Family structure/living arrangement	Children whose single parent has a live-in partner have higher rates of maltreatment overall compared to children living with married biological parents
Family size	Incidence rates are highest for children in the largest families
County metropolitan status	Children from rural counties have a higher rate of overall maltreatment

Preventative measures would need to address the inequities identified below that exist across children regarding developmental adversity.

Evidence of risk for ACEs comes from studies of both children and adults. As described earlier, the NIS-4 (Sedlak et al., 2010) demonstrated that rates of maltreatment for African American children are significantly higher than rates for White/European American and Latin American children. Other risk factors identified in the NIS-4 are highlighted in Table 1.3.

In a recent study of adults (Cronholm et al., 2015), demographic characteristics associated with higher risk for ACEs included adults who reported a race of "other" (versus white); were living with a partner (versus married); were disabled (versus working full-time); younger age; and being separated from one's partner (versus married). Combined with findings from child studies, this evidence has a direct bearing on both preventive interventions and social justice. Primary prevention efforts, for example, include preventing ACEs so that children (especially those with marginalized backgrounds) grow up with less adversity and are less likely to have their own children who are exposed to ACEs (Oral et al., 2016). To address the known racial and ethnic inequities, prevention strategies also need to comprise more resources in place for those children at relatively greatest risk for ACEs (for example, African American and Latin American children). Perhaps most importantly, though, we need to acknowledge and recognize how experiences of racism impact children and their health.

Exposure to Racism as a Developmental Adversity

In today's society, we can no longer discuss trauma and adversity without including racism as a vital topic. In the United States, the total population comprises 38.4% of people of color/non-white (US Census Bureau, 2021). Table 1.4 outlines the major races and ethnicities documented in this most recent census. At its most basic level, racism is the belief that all members of a given race possess characteristics or abilities specific to that race, consequently distinguishing them as supposedly inferior or superior to other races. This erroneous thinking can then lead to racial discrimination in which a person acts for or against an individual or group based on apparent "membership" of that race. Exposure to such behavior is rampant in the United States (and worldwide), with rates of discriminatory treatment of people of color upward to 75%, especially toward non-Latino African Americans (Lee et al., 2019; Woo, 2018).

Although racism is based on a classification system of race as a primarily biological factor, the accepted contemporary view is that race is a social construct (Jones, 2001). Thus, racism occurs at multiple levels of our social ecology (Paradies et al., 2015; Paradies, 2006). The most proximate level is intrinsic to a given individual, who has an internalized worldview of prejudice, attitudes, and beliefs of racism. The next level is interpersonal in nature when racism occurs during interactions between individuals. Lastly, systemic racism is at the level of organizations and institutions, such as governmental bodies, laws, and policies. Regardless of level, however, racism exemplifies the many dimensions of childhood adversity derived from social inequities that have been typically ignored by clinicians and researchers alike (McEwen & Gregerson, 2019).

For our purposes, racism must be viewed and understood as yet another ACE to which children can be exposed. As a distinct adversity, racism in all

Table 1.4 US census data (US Census Bureau, 2021).

Race or ethnicity	Percentage of population (%)
White alone[a]	61.6
Hispanic/Latino	18.7
Black/African American alone	12.4
American Indian/Alaska Native alone	1.1
Asian alone	6.0
Native Hawaiian/Pacific Islander alone	0.2
Some Other Race alone	8.4
Multiracial	10.2

a) Three racial composition concepts were used: race alone, race in combination, and race alone or in combination.

its forms and levels is a stressor that can impact an individual's health and psychosocial functioning (Clark et al., 1999; Mays et al., 2007; Meyer, 2003). The potential chronicity of racism can thus be likened to what we know about children's biobehavioral development when their stress response systems are highly activated for extended durations—a significant wear-and-tear effect on their developing brains and other biological systems with long-term effects on learning, behavior, and health (Forde et al., 2019; Geronimus et al., 2006; McEwen, 2006). This perspective thus indicates that continual coping with discrimination and systemic racism is a potent activator of the stress response (Center on the Developing Child, n.d.).

Summary

Clearly, children can experience a variety of severe adversities. Besides different forms of child abuse and neglect (which, by definition, are perpetrated by parents or other caregivers), other seriously negative experiences count as well, such as the ones identified in the ACE Study (for example, parental impairment), even though they don't meet the threshold definition of *trauma*. Exposure to violence is yet another adversity that requires our attention and that comprises various types (for example, conventional crime, victimization by peers and siblings, witnessing and indirect victimization, and Internet victimization; Finkelhor et al., 2015b). The scientific literature also indicates that inequities exist in which certain children are at increased risk of exposure to ACEs compared to others. Factors identified to distinguish such children include race/ethnicity, sex, age, disability status, school enrollment, and family size. Lastly, racism is a relatively neglected and underappreciated adversity that impacts most non-white children. ACEs are thus collectively vast in number and type and ultimately affect many children regardless. The next section provides an overview of the impact of developmental adversity on developmental processes.

Effects of ACEs on Child Development

Child Abuse and Neglect

The majority of research on the impact of ACEs on child development comes from studies of child abuse and neglect. The effects of such adversity on children's psychosocial development and long-term behavioral health have been well documented. Characteristics of the experience (such as timing, duration, frequency, severity, degree of threat, and relationship to the perpetrator) have been shown to be associated with outcome (Bulik et al., 2001; Keiley et al., 2001; Manly et al., 2001). For example, Navalta et al. (2006) showed that the duration of sexual abuse in females directly relates to the extent of their memory problems. Curiously, although earlier research and clinical lore strongly suggested that children who are traumatized by a parent/caregiver have more severe symptoms than youth who are traumatized by a non-caregiver, more recent findings indicate that abuse by caregivers results in fewer symptoms and problems than abuse perpetrated by a non-caregiving relative (e.g., Kiser et al., 2014).

Consequences of exposure to childhood maltreatment include dysfunctional behaviors, such as conduct problems, oppositional behavior, aggression, and substance use problems (Cicchetti & Handley, 2019; Fergusson et al., 1996; Schuck & Widom, 2001). The former externalizing behavior problems have been hypothesized to link alcohol use in adolescents with maltreatment and violence during childhood (Cornelius et al., 2016; Proctor et al., 2017). Exposure to child abuse and neglect also leads to an increased risk for later mental health problems, including depression, suicide, anxiety disorder, somatization disorders, and post-traumatic stress disorder (PTSD) (Brown et al., 1999; Fergusson et al., 1996; Fergusson & Lynskey, 1997; Lansford et al., 2002). In general, interpersonal trauma (such as child maltreatment) is much more likely to lead to PTSD than non-interpersonal trauma (Alisic et al., 2014). Emerging research indicates that earlier adversity more strongly influences anxiety, mood, and anhedonia, whereas relatively later adversity has greater effects on externalizing behavior problems (Andersen, 2015). Associations with psychopathology during adulthood are independent of other associated environmental adversities (Brown et al., 1999; Fergusson et al., 1996).

Both commonalities and distinctions exist in the effects of maltreatment across abuse types. Physical abuse, for example, is associated with symptoms of depression, emotional distress, and suicidal ideation (Green, 1988; Waldrop et al., 2007) as well as increased risk of developing a substance use disorder in adolescence (Kilpatrick et al., 2003). Sexual abuse-specific symptoms include PTSD, dissociation, depression, and sexual problems (for a comprehensive review, see Sanjeevi et al., 2018). Emotional abuse, in contrast, is particularly associated with aggressive behavior, especially when the abuse is developmentally early and severe (Manly et al., 2001) or primarily verbal (Vissing et al., 1991). Children who have been neglected also exhibit high levels of aggression (de Paúl & Arruabarrena, 1995; Kaufman & Cicchetti, 1989; Kotch et al., 2008).

The clinical picture becomes complex when children experience multiple incidents and forms of child abuse and neglect or ACEs in general (Finkelhor et al., 2007). Generally, a dose-response relationship exists whereby: (a) a certain minimal number of exposures is necessary for the development of an adverse outcome, such as persistent internalizing or externalizing disorders; and (b) the greater the number of forms of ACEs, the more severe the subsequent problems and the greater the amount of utilization of psychiatric care

(Caspi et al., 2003; Edwards et al., 2003; Putnam et al., 2013; Teicher et al., 2006).

Child maltreatment is associated with a host of neurocognitive deficits and related psychosocial impairment. Poor school performance is tied to exposure to child abuse and neglect (Crozier & Barth, 2005; Trocme & Caunce, 1995; Veltman & Browne, 2001), such as problems with grades, test scores, and school absences as well as later dropout (Leiter & Johnsen, 1994). Children who have been neglected exhibit lower performance scores in reading and math, lower grades, and higher levels of suspensions, disciplinary referrals, grade repetitions, dropouts, absences, and special education involvement (Eckenrode et al., 1993; Kendall-Tackett & Eckenrode, 1996; Leiter & Johnsen, 1997; Wodarski et al., 1990). Such scholastic deficiencies are associated with problems in auditory attention, flexibility, response inhibition, and visual-motor integration (Nolin & Ethier, 2007). In addition, intelligence deficits have been reported across types of child maltreatment (Malinosky-Rummell & Hansen, 1993; Veltman & Browne, 2001), although other characteristics of the adversity influence the extent of the problems, such as duration, severity, and timing during development (Kavanaugh et al., 2017), as well as other environmental factors (Ayoub et al., 2006). Childhood maltreatment, however, has not been consistently shown to change basic memory processes nor influence the encoding, storing, and recall of memories (Goodman et al., 2010; Howe et al., 2006). Future studies are needed, though to flesh out potentially important factors that may moderate or mediate maltreatment effects on memory; for example, forms of abuse or neglect experienced, the presence of trauma and/or dissociative symptoms, parenting style, and the type of stimuli to be recalled (Dalgleish et al., 2005; Navalta, 2011).

Developmental adversity has definitively been shown to be associated with alterations in brain structure and function, systemic inflammation, and circuits that regulate endocrine, behavioral, immune, and autonomic responses to stress (for recent comprehensive reviews, see Lippard & Nemeroff, 2020; Nemeroff, 2016; Teicher & Samson, 2016). Specific structural changes have been documented in the following brain regions: anterior cingulate cortex; dorsolateral prefrontal and orbitofrontal cortex; corpus callosum; and adult hippocampus. Functional imaging studies have consistently shown an enhanced response of the amygdala to emotional faces and a diminished response of the ventral striatum to anticipated rewards. Specific ACEs also seem to selectively target sensory systems and pathways that convey and process the adverse experience, which indicates that the type of adversity does matter. Exposure to severe parental verbal abuse, for example, is related to gray matter volume changes in the left auditory cortex as well as decreased stability of a specific language pathway known as the left arcuate fasciculus (Choi et al., 2009; Tomoda et al., 2011). In addition, the impact of ACEs is partly dependent on the timing of exposure and the child's sex, such as ACEs being associated with a relatively smaller corpus callosum and hippocampus in boys than girls. Overall, these brain regions and pathways underlie the regulation of detecting threat/danger and anticipating reward (Teicher & Samson, 2016), and the known impact of ACEs on brain development supports the evolution-framed neurodevelopmental model articulated by Navalta et al. (2008b), which includes the following four postulates:

1) The brain goes through one or more sensitive periods in postnatal life when exposure to high levels of stress hormones selects for an alternative pathway of neurodevelopment;
2) The ensuing developmental trajectory is an adaptive one;
3) Exposure to corticosteroids is a keystone element in organizing the brain to develop in this manner; and
4) Disparate brain systems are affected by different types of ACEs, particularly the primary and secondary sensory systems that may be especially involved in perceiving or recalling the adversities.

ACEs and Health Disorders

Generally speaking, a health *problem* gets diagnosed as a health *disorder* when functional impairment or clinical distress is established. Impairment is present whenever symptoms interfere with the individual's participation in expected activities, according to the World Health Organization (2001). In children, behavioral health disorders associated with ACEs include PTSD, acute stress disorder (ASD), depressive disorders, prolonged grief disorder, anxiety disorders, and externalizing disorders (Alisic et al., 2020). The ACE Study demonstrated that behavioral health disorders in adults with histories of developmental adversity are many and varied, such as substance use disorder, depressive disorders, psychotic disorders, and impulse control disorders (Felitti et al., 1998; Whitfield et al., 2005), which have been validated by replication studies (e.g., Putnam et al., 2013). Physical health problems were also elucidated in the ACE Study, including ischemic heart disease, cancer, chronic lung disease, skeletal fractures, and liver disease (Felitti et al., 1998).

Perhaps most troublesome are findings indicating that poor physical health outcomes can be present well before adulthood (Flaherty et al., 2013; Layne et al., 2014). For example, a graded relationship was found between ACEs and any health problem (e.g., poor health, illness requiring a doctor, somatic concerns) by 14 years of age in a sample of children with reported or at risk for abuse and neglect (Flaherty et al., 2013). Similarly, less school engagement and more chronic disease were documented among children with ACEs in the 2011–2012 National Survey of Children's Health (Bethell et al., 2014). Headaches, migraines, and stomachaches have been specifically tied to exposure to community and interpersonal violence or disaster during childhood (Bailey et al., 2005; Stensland et al., 2014) as well as chronic pain and musculoskeletal problems (Dirkzwager et al., 2006; Dorn et al., 2008). Although the interplay between physical and behavioral health problems associated with ACEs isn't fully understood, such somatic health problems can influence the child's ability to attend school, participate in leisure activities, and engage in social relationships (Alisic et al., 2020)—hallmarks of the World Health Organization's (2001) definition of impairment.

Developmental Trauma Disorder: A Proposed Diagnosis with Emergent Scientific Validity

Children and adolescents exposed to developmental adversity often experience multiple problems simultaneously, especially when ACEs are numerous or repeated (Copeland et al., 2007). However, the breadth of negative consequences has resulted in the absence of a thorough understanding and explanation of the connection between the children's life histories and their biobehavioral development (D'Andrea et al., 2012; McLaughlin, 2016). For adults (and evidently applicable to children and adolescents), the most recent and regarded attempt at a broader category of trauma-related psychopathology is the diagnosis of complex PTSD in the International Classification of Diseases 11th Revision (World Health Organization, 2018). The "complex" aspect of this new diagnosis is disturbances in self-organization, which are labeled as affect dysregulation, negative self-concept, and interpersonal problems. Similarly, the proposed diagnosis, Developmental Trauma Disorder (DTD), was created to capture these same problems, although the diagnosis wasn't included in DSM-5 (American Psychiatric Association, 2013a) allegedly due to insufficient empirical support (Schmid et al., 2013).

van der Kolk et al. (2009) argued in the original proposal for DTD that a new diagnosis is needed to capture the clinical presentations of children and adolescents exposed to chronic interpersonal trauma because the PTSD diagnosis (and all other diagnoses in DSM) does not truly represent the clinical picture of the youth. As a result, the children receive no diagnosis or multiple unrelated diagnoses (D'Andrea et al., 2012). van der Kolk et al. (2009) also highlighted the fact that the PTSD diagnosis at that time (i.e., DSM-IV-TR; American Psychiatric Association, 2000) was developmentally insensitive (DSM-5 now has a "preschool" subtype for post-traumatic stress symptoms).

A study by Spinazzola et al. (2005) illustrates the characteristics of the children regarding their exposure to ACEs and their symptomatology. Across a sample of 1,699 children receiving trauma-focused treatment at sites of the National Child Traumatic Stress Network, almost 80% of them had been exposed to multiple and/or prolonged interpersonal trauma (modal number of exposure types = 3). While less than 25% met diagnostic criteria for PTSD, at least 50% had significant disturbances in emotion regulation, attention/concentration, self-image, impulse control, aggression, and risk-taking behavior. Follow-up studies have validated these findings and demonstrated that this spectrum of specific symptoms should be the area of focus for a more thorough understanding and explanation of the connection between the children's life histories and their biobehavioral development rather than merely emphasizing traditional psychiatric categorizations (D'Andrea et al., 2012; Ford et al., 2013).

Since the original proposal of DTD (van der Kolk et al., 2009), further scientific support for the diagnosis has emerged. Children who've been chronically maltreated, exposed to violence, or experienced caregiving disruptions, for example, are more likely than children without such adversity histories to meet the criteria for DTD (Stolbach et al., 2013). Compared to the diagnosis of PTSD, DTD is seen by professionals as having comparable clinical utility, being distinct (and not simply a more severe form nor subtype of PTSD), and having a similar or poorer response to science-based treatments (DePierro et al., 2019; Ford et al., 2013). Together, this combined evidence reinforces the DTD diagnosis as a distinct syndrome (DePierro et al., 2019), although the clinical presentation can often include PTSD and other behavioral health disorders as co-occurring conditions (Ford et al., 2018; van Der Kolk et al., 2019).

Effects of ACEs on the Family

By definition, childhood is a developmental stage when the individual is dependent on adults for basic necessities for survival, such as food, clothing, and shelter. Adult caregivers are also needed for the child to develop along expected, typical developmental trajectories across all areas of functioning—biologically, psychologically, socially, and culturally/contextually. However, not only does developmental adversity negatively impact a given child, but ACEs can also affect the parents, other family members, and broader caregiving systems (Galano & Graham-Bermann, 2019; NCTSN Core Curriculum on Childhood Trauma Task Force, 2012). The most immediate and proximal system is the family, although schools and communities are integral systems as well. Typically, where a child lives day-to-day includes and defines who that child's family is, such as parents, stepparents, and siblings (biological and "step"). Extended family members can also be part of the picture (grandparents, aunts, uncles, cousins) and families, in general, can differ based on composition, for example, single-parent, adoptive, divorced, "step," multigenerational, and families with parents who have varied gender identities and sexual orientations (Galano & Graham-Bermann, 2019).

Because children don't live in a vacuum but instead inhabit families, what impacts them can also directly or indirectly affect other family members, including exposure to trauma and adversity. The influence of such experiences on families has perhaps been best understood through the lens of systems theory (Bronfenbrenner, 1979; Gelles & Maynard, 1987; Howes et al., 2000; Patterson, 1991; Shochet & Dadds, 1997). Two major principles of the theory are the following: (a) an event or experience that affects one family member influences the entire family system; and (b) all systems strive to maintain balance or homeostasis. Accordingly, ACEs can influence the family system in one or more of the following ways: (a) simultaneous exposure of all family members to the same event or experience; (b) vicarious trauma from an exposed family member to others in the family; (c) intrafamilial trauma in which a family member is the perpetrator; and (d) secondary stress when a child's trauma-related symptoms disrupt family functioning (Collins et al., 2011). When adversely affected as such, the family works toward regaining any balance that was consequently lost, according to systems theory.

In general, developmental adversity can significantly impact family and extended caregiving systems and thus result in serious disruptions in caregiver-child interactions and attachment relationships (NCTSN Core Curriculum on Childhood Trauma Task Force, 2012). Not surprisingly, if parents are negatively affected by their children's exposure to ACEs (or have histories of health-related problems or other struggles), their parenting behaviors may change, including how they respond to their children's reactions and responses to trauma and adversity. Elevated parenting stress, for example, has been shown to be uniquely predicted by exposure to multiple ACEs as well as associated with children's trauma-related symptoms (Hickman et al., 2013; Salloum et al., 2015). Exposure to intimate partner violence is associated with the potential to perpetrate child abuse, use of physical discipline, inconsistent discipline, and restrictive/punitive parenting, particularly in mothers of children exposed to such adversity (Cohen et al., 2008; Greene et al., 2018; Symes et al., 2016). Furthermore, the relationship between adults in the family as well as ones among siblings can all be compromised to the point when interactions become overburdened. Such strain can thus lead to problems in communicating, regulating emotions, and remaining close that, in turn, increases the chances for conflict, separation, or even interpersonal violence (Collins et al., 2011; Galano & Graham-Bermann, 2019).

Dysregulation of Emotions and Related Behaviors

Affective (emotional) and physiological dysregulation is one of the main symptom domains in the present diagnostic conceptualization of DTD (the others being attentional and behavioral dysregulation, self and relational dysregulation, and at least some classic PTSD symptoms; Ford et al., 2018). In contrast, when children follow a typical developmental path that is not disrupted by ACEs, they eventually learn how to adequately monitor, evaluate, and modify their emotions—in other words, regulate their emotions to accomplish their goals or to meet the demands of the present environment (Thompson, 1994). Known as emotion regulation, this capacity is an adaptive, regulatory process vital for healthy psychosocial development and a critical life skill that predicts positive long-term outcomes. If children endure developmental adversity, however, they can end up having problems in effectively regulating their emotions, that is, experience emotion dysregulation. At less severe levels, emotion dysregulation is typically observed as internalizing symptoms (for example, depressive, eating, or anxiety disorders), whereas externalizing behavior problems are present when emotion dysregulation is relatively more severe, such as self-injury, aggression, substance use, and sexual behavior (D'Andrea et al., 2012; Ford et al., 2013). In sum, problems in emotion regulation have been identified as a central feature of children impacted by ACEs, in particular the regulation of negative emotions, such as anxiety, fear, and anger.

Mechanistically, emotion dysregulation has been hypothesized as a central developmental mechanism linking ACEs with psychopathology and results from deficient down-regulation of brain systems associated with emotional responding (Dvir et al., 2014; Heleniak et al., 2016; Maughan & Cicchetti, 2002; McLaughlin et al., 2015). Converging evidence indicates that exposure to ACEs is associated with heightened reactivity to negative emotional cues (in other words, heightened perception of threat or danger). Examples of this increased reactivity include biased attention toward potential threats or danger in the environment, greater neurobiological and subjective responses to negative emotional cues, and a unique pattern of the nervous system that regulates involuntary physiologic processes, including heart rate, blood pressure, respiration, digestion, and sexual arousal (Heleniak et al., 2016; McLaughlin et al., 2014, 2015; Pollak et al., 2005; Shackman et al., 2007). Such elevated emotional reactivity makes emotion regulation more difficult for children exposed to ACEs and is associated with areas of the prefrontal cortex involved in effortful control (McLaughlin et al., 2015). Emotion dysregulation may also be due, in part, to its reliance on executive function, which is negatively impacted by developmental adversity as well (Cowell et al., 2015; Kavanaugh & Holler, 2015; Skowron et al., 2014). The fact that the capacity for emotion regulation increases developmentally, however, implies that children can learn and improve their ability to regulate emotions. Enhancing emotion regulation strategies in children impacted by adversity is known to reduce clinical symptoms and improve psychosocial functioning (Riley et al., 2017). Consequently, the Trauma-Informed Parenting Program (*TIP^s for Clinicians*) was uniquely developed to capitalize on the social influence that parents have on their children's emotion regulation (Martin & Ochsner, 2016).

Overview of the Parent Training Program: From Emotion Dysregulation to Emotion Regulation

The clinical and scientific rationale for the *Trauma-Informed Parenting Program (TIP^s for Clinicians)* is based on the following four premises:

1) Emotion dysregulation is a core problem cluster within a spectrum of clinical problems observed in adversity-affected children
2) Emotion dysregulation is hypothesized to be a central developmental mechanism linking developmental adversity with psychopathology
3) Emotion regulation development is largely dependent on how parents respond to their children's emotions; and
4) Parent training is a scientifically well-established intervention approach for childhood behavior problems.

As previously reviewed, systems theory has been vital in helping to understand the impact of trauma and adversity on children and families. Interventions targeted at the systems level are likewise essential for children who've been exposed to ACEs. The foundation for *TIP^s* thus capitalizes on the most influential people within the system in closest proximity, the children's parent(s).

One useful framework to best understand *TIP^s* comes from the science-based treatment, Trauma Systems Therapy (TST; Navalta et al., 2013; Saxe et al., 2007). The transactions between a child and parent are called the *trauma system* in TST. As defined, the trauma system comprises two components: (a) a child who exhibits emotion dysregulation; and (b) a social environment that is challenged in containing this dysregulation. In *TIP^s*, the parent(s) is the targeted social environment who can help enhance their child's emotion regulation in their role as a vital adult caregiver. Not surprisingly, other trauma-focused, systems-oriented interventions also aim to improve children's emotion regulation skills, including Attachment, Regulation, and Competency (ARC; Blaustein & Kinniburgh, 2010). Skill-building approaches teach children adaptive ways of regulating their negative emotions to ultimately improve adjustment (Hannesdóttir & Ollendick, 2017).

Emotion regulation develops as a function of both intrinsic and extrinsic processes, including parents (Eisenberg et al., 2010; Stegge & Terwogt, 2007; Thompson & Goodman, 2010) as well as social, interpersonal, and cultural factors (Riediger & Klipker, 2014; Thompson & Goodman, 2010). Neurobiological advances beginning in middle childhood (for example, development of executive functions) enable greater awareness and management of emotion (Lane et al., 1990). Some of the most common strategies that children use to regulate emotions are the following: emotional expression, emotional suppression, problem-solving, cognitive reappraisal, distraction, acceptance, avoidance, wishful thinking, denial, emotional modulation, the unregulated release of emotions, and humor (Compas et al., 2017). At its most fundamental level, *TIP^s* guides clinicians to train parents to (a) help their children recognize when they move from emotional states of regulation to dysregulation; and (b) teach their children specific coping and emotion identification/understanding skills.

TIP^s also benefits from the scientific advances of parent training models for the treatment of child behavioral health problems. These interventions have been most successful for disruptive behavior problems in particular (Chorpita et al., 2011; Coates et al., 2015), although some empirical support exists for internalizing symptoms (Eckshtain et al., 2017; Gonzalez & Jones, 2016). The models all share the following core elements (Shaffer et al., 2001):

1) Focus more on parents than the child
2) Move from an emphasis on antisocial behavior to prosocial behavior
3) Teach parents to identify, define, and record child behavior
4) Instruct parents in social learning principles
5) Teach new parenting skills via didactic instruction, modeling, role-playing, and practicing with the child
6) Discuss ways to maximize generalization of skills from the clinic to the home
7) Address parental, family, and community risk factors that may interfere with the acquisition or maintenance of new parenting skills and adaptive child behavior

In contrast, *TIP^s* is unique in that the treatment doesn't just teach parents how to increase desirable child behavior and decrease undesirable behavior. Rather, *TIP^s* targets the emotion regulation problems that children impacted by developmental adversity have. Emotion dysregulation is hypothesized to be a central mechanism that links exposure to ACEs to later behavioral health problems, as described earlier in this chapter. Because the problems can be many and varied, an alternative, albeit consistent, premise is that such dysregulation is a transdiagnostic risk factor or pathway for multiple behavioral health conditions (Werner & Gross, 2010). This transdiagnostic perspective has a direct bearing on *TIP^s* in that the focus of treatment isn't on the differing psychopathological outcomes that the children can have but rather on an underlying process for the onset and maintenance of clinical problems (Chu, 2012). For our purposes, emotion dysregulation is that very process that *TIP^s* targets. This newer therapeutic strategy has been called the *core dysfunction approach* (Marchette & Weisz, 2017). At its core, *TIP^s* directly addresses the children's emotion dysregulation that, in turn, leads to improvements in their behavioral health.

TIP^s is a unique intervention created for behavioral healthcare providers that centers on training or teaching parents to help their children who are having problems regulating their emotions. Although the treatment is focused on helping children exposed to developmental adversity and the resulting emotion dysregulation, many of the tools found in this manual are also applicable to use with parents who have children with problems in regulating their emotions that are not related to ACEs, for example, children diagnosed with Oppositional Defiant Disorder who experience high levels of frustration and anger.

Emotion dysregulation is a fundamental problem for children who have been exposed to developmental adversity. Such dysregulation typically leads to internalizing symptoms when the problem is less severe but results in highly disruptive and potentially risky or dangerous behavior when the dysregulation is more problematic. *TIP^s* provides real-world, practical strategies and techniques for clinicians to train parents to address their children's emotion dysregulation and related behavior problems. The negative emotions that the children experience when dysregulated are presumed to be elicited by trauma reminders. In other words, unique cues, stimuli, or triggers that are associated with the children's trauma memories are what bring about these negative emotional states. When sufficiently elevated, the emotions interfere with the child's ability to engage in their immediate surroundings and participate in the activity at hand. The child thus doesn't have the internal resources to turn things around and re-engage with their environment. Such circumstances are the very ones in which parents (or other adult caregivers in close proximity) have the opportunity to intervene to help the child get back to a regulated state. *TIP^s* provides a trauma-informed parent training model for parents to develop and possess the tools necessary to teach their children how to effectively regulate their emotions in their daily lives. Such an outcome aligns with the concept of *resilience* as defined by Southwick et al. (2014)—"healthy, adaptive, or integrated positive functioning over the passage of time in the aftermath of adversity."

2

Clinical Assessment

> At the end of this chapter, you will be able to:
>
> - Understand a trauma-informed strategy for assessment
> - Describe how an accurate and comprehensive assessment is the first step toward clinical understanding
> - Summarize a multi-method, multi-informant approach to assessing children and their families
> - Conduct an assessment of an episode of emotion dysregulation

"Assess to Understand"

Several years ago, this manual's author created a mantra as a simple guide to help his graduate students navigate the early phases of treatment: *"Assess to understand before you intervene."* In essence, this brief phrase captures the three main therapeutic activities sequentially conducted by clinicians—assessment, case conceptualization, and intervention. Clinically indicated treatments and interventions can be recommended only after an accurate and comprehensive clinical understanding of a child is achieved. For our purposes, this knowledge is called case conceptualization, which will be covered in detail in Chapter 3. Likewise, the understanding of a child's clinical symptoms and problems is best achieved by conducting a thorough yet focused assessment. Such an assessment is thus required to begin the process of helping children who've been exposed to developmental adversity.

Based on the information presented in Chapter 1, we know that children can be exposed to many and varied adversities. Childhood can be filled with such encounters, whether these experiences are traumatic, sub-threshold traumatic, or significantly adverse/stressful. Unfortunately, we also know that the more children have these occurrences, the more the risk their biopsychosocial

Trauma-Informed Parenting Program: TIP^s for Clinicians to Train Parents of Children Impacted by Trauma & Adversity, First Edition. Carryl P. Navalta.
© 2022 John Wiley & Sons, Inc. Published 2022 by John Wiley & Sons, Inc.
Companion Website: www.wiley.com/go/navalta/tipsforclinicians

development goes awry. At its worst, the child's brain development will have an abnormal trajectory associated with behavioral health problems, functional impairment, and possibly distress as well. These children are the ones who are at a critical point regarding identification and assessment (Berliner et al., 2020).

Methods and Domains of Assessment

The range of exposure to developmental adversity and resulting behavioral health problems exemplifies how assessments should be constructed sensitively to capture patterns of co-occurrence of symptoms and contextual variations (De Los Reyes et al., 2018). Fortunately, clinicians can choose from several assessment activities to strategically gather the clinical information required to arrive at an adequate case conceptualization. Such undertakings include one or more of the following:

- Use of diagnostic categories to describe child problems and symptoms (e.g., DSM-5; ICD-11)
- Use of standardized and non-standardized psychological instruments and educational tests
- Clinical interview
- Behavioral observations
- Analysis of case records
- Gathering information from significant others, such as parents and teachers

Although clinicians may be tempted to take a minimalist approach to assessment due to various reasons (e.g., time constraints) and choose to use a couple (or perhaps only one) of the activities above, they need to remember that no gold standard measure exists to quantify child behavioral health problems, including symptoms associated with exposure to adverse childhood experiences (ACEs). A vital, related fact is that no single measure can comprehensively index therapeutic change, progress, or improvement. Consequently, reliable and valid assessments need to comprise multiple informants and measurement methods (De Los Reyes et al., 2015).

In general, parents of children exposed to developmental adversity and other caregivers (including teachers when possible) should be directly included in the assessment. Based on their observations and interactions with their children in varied activities, events, and situations, they can provide important historical information (e.g., pre-adversity functioning, a timeline of symptom presentation), family functioning details (e.g., family reaction and adaptation to the trauma), and collateral information on the child's symptomatology (Berliner et al., 2020). Although the information gathered from parents may be discrepant from data collected from their children (Achenbach et al., 1987; De Los Reyes et al., 2015), such divergent findings may turn out to be clinically useful because they can occur for systematic reasons corresponding to a child's differing clinical presentations, such as when a parent is supporting the child's emotion regulation at home versus a teacher in the classroom (De Los Reyes et al., 2018).

Rating Scales

The use of rating scales is an integral assessment method for clinicians. Contemporary scales typically have a high level of standardization such that the procedures for administering them are concrete and easy to follow. Other important features of rating scales include the following: (a) the sample(s) of individuals used in the development of the measure; (b) its reliability and validity; (c) sensitivity and specificity; (d) the presence of cutoff scores; and (e) efficiency of use. Depending on the purpose of a given scale, the developers may have used a non-clinical sample, clinical sample, and/or a normative sample to make comparisons. Therefore, clinicians need to know beforehand some relevant information about their child client to decide what sample(s) is most pertinent. Clinicians are also recommended to use instruments that are both reliable (i.e., consistent) and valid, which means that the scale truly measures the process or construct in question. One example is construct validity, in which the soundness of the tool depends on the identification and creation of the items comprised in the scale. In addition, rating scales need to be sensitive to accurately identifying that the problem exists ("true positive") as well as specific in identifying when the problem isn't present ("true negative"). Such a boundary occurs when measures have operational cutoff scores to determine whether the problem is present or not. Lastly, clinicians should choose scales that can be completed quickly and scored easily.

Exposure to Developmental Adversity

Checklists that include a trauma and adversity screen and an assessment of post-traumatic stress symptoms are readily available. An example is the Child Trauma Screen (Lang & Connell, 2017), a brief, psychometrically solid screener in the public domain that comprises just four items. More comprehensive measures include the Child and Adolescent Trauma Screen (Sachser et al., 2017), Child PTSD Symptom Scale for DSM-5 (Foa et al., 2018), and the UCLA PTSD Reaction Index (Kaplow et al., 2020). The Trauma Event Screening Inventory (Choi et al., 2019) should be considered when gathering detailed information about exposure across multiple ACEs.

One crucial ACE that the instruments mentioned above fail to cover is racism and racial discrimination exposure. The idea of racism as a unique stressor is not new. For example, Clark et al. (1999) proposed a model in which an environmental stimulus can be perceived as racist—a trigger signaling

(a) antagonism toward an individual or group based on group membership; and (b) inferiority to another race or races. Exposure to such stimulation then results in exaggerated psychological and physiological stress responses, which over time influence health outcomes. Not surprisingly, exposure to racism is associated with many socioemotional, behavioral, and academic problems. Children exposed to racism, for example, have an increased risk for developing depression, anxiety, anger, and aggression problems (Pachter & Coll, 2009; Priest et al., 2013), whereas teenagers are more prone to problems with substance use, sexual behavior, and peer affiliations (Benner et al., 2018). Through a systems lens, the Developmental and Ecological Model of Youth Racial Trauma (DEMYth-RT) provides an ecological framework for how exposure to racism can impact family and community systems within the child's environment and how these systems are integral to the interpretation and management of racism by children as a unique developmental adversity. Assessing for exposure to racism and addressing its impact on the health and well-being of children and adolescents are thus imperative (Trent et al., 2019).

Fortunately, a psychometric tool is available that was specifically created to assess for exposure to racism—Perceptions of Racism in Children and Youth (PRaCY; Pachter et al., 2010). The PRaCY is a reliable and valid self-report instrument that measures perceptions of racism and discrimination in children and youth aged 8–18 years with diverse racial and ethnic backgrounds and identities. Two short versions of the scale exist (the second contains an additional response category for the frequency of racist events). An extended version is also available that includes response categories for frequency, attribution, emotional response, and coping response to racist events.

Although created for use with adults, the UConn Racial/ Ethnic Stress & Trauma Survey (UnRESTS; Williams et al., 2018) can be used as a guide for clinicians to ask further questions regarding experiences of racism that are less overt or direct. For example, one section of the instrument focuses on ascertaining whether the person has been impacted by racism due to an experience of a loved one or someone close to them. Another area of inquiry is exposure to *vicarious* racism—racism resulting from learning about an incident that involved someone not personally known to the individual. Lastly, experiences of subtle or covert racism are queried. Examples include the following acts: (a) microassaults: "explicit racial derogation(s) characterized primarily by a verbal or nonverbal attack meant to hurt the intended victim through name-calling, avoidant behavior, or purposeful discriminatory actions" (Sue et al., 2007, p. 277); (b) microinsults: barbs and put-downs that impart negative or even humiliating messages to recipients; and (c) microinvalidations: acts that "exclude, negate, or nullify the psychological thoughts, feelings, or experiential reality of a person of color" (Sue et al., 2007, p. 274). Although beyond the scope of this chapter (and more challenging to assess), the existence of systemic racism must be at the very least acknowledged if not outright directly measured if the clinician suspects that a child has been exposed to such adversity, especially in a sustained manner. This form of racism occurs, as the name implies, in organizations and institutions, such as governmental bodies, laws, and policies.

With the onset of the COVID-19 pandemic, we now must examine how this mass or collective adversity has played out in the lives of *all* children and families with whom we work. Our efforts should be grounded on the assumption that everyone has been negatively impacted in some way. Thus, our assessments need to include exposure to stress associated with the pandemic and its aftermath. Related to consequences such as schools shutting down and withdrawal from social life and outdoor activities, many families have experienced significant socio-emotional stress (and financial stress, too) due to the pandemic (Phelps & Sperry, 2020). In addition, learning remotely and "doing school" from home have had their unique challenges—not the least of which has been whether children have had consistent and adequate-quality internet access. Through a biopsychosocial lens, de Figueiredo et al. (2021) emphasized that the withdrawal from social life, daily activities, and in-person learning at school, combined with fear, anxiety, and unpredictability, increase the risk for children to develop behavioral health problems, even for those who do not have such histories.

Given that the COVID-19 pandemic is a relatively new and evolving public health crisis, only a small number of measures is available to assess children's exposure to pandemic-related stressors. The Coronavirus Impact Scale (Stoddard et al., 2021) is an 11-item self-report scale that an adult family member can complete. Items are rated on a four-point Likert scale and include the following domains: routines, income/employment, access (food, healthcare, social supports), stress, and exposure to/knowledge of family members or close friends with COVID-19. The COVID-19 Exposure and Family Impact Scales (CEFIS; Kazak et al., 2021) were developed to assess exposure to potentially traumatic aspects of COVID-19 and the impact of the pandemic on the family. Completed by caregivers, the CEFIS includes items covering areas such as "stay at home" order, the closing of schools/childcare centers, disruption of children's education, and inability to visit or care for family members.

Assessment of Symptomatology
Many questionnaires and checklists are available to assess trauma-related symptoms and problems—many of which are free and in the public domain—and determine if symptoms are clinically significant. Because the child doesn't have to discuss exposure to ACEs with the clinician, questionnaires can help avoid assessment-related distress. Depending on the

assessment questions, rating scales may need to be chosen based on whether the tools include the most updated diagnostic criteria (e.g., DSM-5) and symptomatology that is typical for the developmental stage of the child who is being assessed (Briggs et al., 2014). Clinicians also need to be mindful of the limitations of these types of instruments, which include the following: (a) required minimum reading comprehension level; (b) risk of incorrect scoring or interpreting; (c) few opportunities for children to ask questions or have the meaning of questionnaire items clarified; (d) risk of measurement error/inaccuracy; (e) cutoff scores that aren't relevant to the child due to the uniqueness of the sample(s) used to create the measures; and (f) risk of the child becoming upset by completing a questionnaire (Berliner et al., 2020).

Regardless of the limitations mentioned above, questionnaires and checklists should be strongly considered when the need to assess for exposure to developmental adversity and consequent symptomatology exists. Table 2.1 outlines many of the currently available measures.

Table 2.1 Rating scales to assess exposure to ACEs and related symptoms.

Questionnaire	Respondent	Age Range (Years)
Child Revised Impact of Events Scale (Perrin et al., 2005)	Child	8–18
Child Stress Disorders Checklist ASD/PTSD (Saxe et al., 2003)	Parent	5–17
Child Stress Disorders Checklist—Short Form (Bosquet Enlow et al., 2010)	Parent	6–18
Child Trauma Screen (Lang & Connell, 2017)	Child, Parent	3–18
Pediatric Emotional Distress Scale (Saylor et al., 1999)	Parent	2–10
Trauma Symptom Checklist for Children (Briere, 1996)	Child	8–16
Trauma Symptom Checklist for Young Children (Briere et al., 2001)	Parent	3–12
Young Child PTSD Screen (Scheeringa & Haslett, 2010)	Parent	3–6
Child Trauma Screening Questionnaire (Kenardy et al., 2006)	Child	7–16
Acute Stress Checklist for Children (Kassam-Adams, 2006)	Child	8–17
Child and Adolescent Trauma Screen (Sachser et al., 2017)	Child, Parent	3–17
Child PTSD Symptom Scale for DSM-5 (Foa et al., 2018)	Child	8–18
UCLA PTSD Reaction Index (Kaplow et al., 2020)	Child, Parent	7–18
My Worst Experiences Survey (National Center for Study of Corporal Punishment and Alternatives in Schools, 1992)	Child	9–18
Parent Report of Child's Reaction to Stress (Fletcher, 1996b)	Parent	Not Applicable

Clinical Interview

Clinical interviews are a primary way that clinicians gather information relevant to the domains of interest. Based on their background, experience, and expertise, clinicians typically conduct interviews by asking questions in an unstructured format. This process allows clinicians to tailor their interviews to their clients/patients and includes an easy, informal recording of responses. The following domains are usually covered in an unstructured interview for children:

- Information related to the referral problem
- Home environment and family relationships
- Friendships and peer interactions
- School
- Activities and interests
- Self-awareness and emotional experiences

However, several limitations are present with unstructured interviews. For example, no standardized areas of inquiry are included, which may lead to the omission of vital information on symptomatology, thereby increasing the chances of making incorrect diagnoses. Therefore, more standardized interviews should be considered because of their increased reliability and validity.

Two types of such interviews exist, semi-structured and structured. Semi-structured interviews comprise a standardized set of questions with added probes that can be used based on clinical judgment. Clinicians can also go "off script" and ask follow-up questions for clarification or additional information. Although these interviews arguably have greater reliability and validity than unstructured ones, the level of improvement is questionable. In contrast, structured interviews have the greatest psychometric properties, and most are created for clinicians to make differential diagnoses. Such interviews include the following characteristics: (a) a formal set of questions and areas of inquiry; (b) standardized administration; and (c) a formal method for rating responses. However, structured interviews limit the variability of the client's clinical presentations, require extensive training for administration, and may omit important information about the client's functioning because of the interview's exclusive focus on diagnostic criteria. Regardless of these shortcomings, both semi-structured and structured interviews are key components of the assessment process.

Several standardized, trauma-specific clinical interviews are available to clinicians (Berliner et al., 2020). These psychometric tools comprise the Clinician-Administered PTSD Scale for DSM-5—Child/Adolescent Version (Pynoos et al., 2015), Child PTSD Symptom Scale for DSM-5 (Foa et al., 2018), Children's Posttraumatic Stress Disorder Inventory (Saigh et al., 2000),

Child PTSD Reaction Index (Frederick et al., 1992), Childhood PTSD Interview (Fletcher, 1996a), and Children's Impact of Traumatic Events Scale-Revised (Chaffin & Shultz, 2001). In addition, interviews that cover a range of diagnostic domains, including PTSD, exist, such as the Anxiety Disorders Interview Schedule (Silverman & Albano, 1996), Kiddie Schedule for Affective Disorders and Schizophrenia (Kaufman et al., 1997), and Diagnostic Infant and Preschool Assessment (Scheeringa & Haslett, 2010).

Before moving on to the assessment of emotion and emotion regulation, processes or factors that contribute to maintaining symptoms and problems need to be acknowledged. As described in Chapter 3 on case conceptualization, the third of the *3 Ps* or *Triple Ps* is known as **P**erpetuating factors, which can be internal or external to the individual. For our purposes, one intrinsic process to account for is various cognitions that a child may have (for example, thoughts, ideas, and beliefs), and a potential extrinsic variable is parental behavior and functioning. Fortunately, measures are available to assess these possible perpetuating factors, including the Child Post-Traumatic Cognitions Inventory (Meiser-Stedman et al., 2009), Parent Trauma Response Questionnaire (Williamson et al., 2018), and Thinking about Recovery Scale (Schilpzand et al., 2018). By definition, if these factors are not identified and diminished/eliminated, the child will continue to experience emotional and behavioral problems.

When do we as clinicians know when a developmental process isn't taking its expected course? From the framework of developmental psychopathology, "normal," "average," or "typical" processes need to be firmly established before "abnormal," "non-average," or "atypical" ones (e.g., symptomatology, dysfunction, dysregulation) can be understood and identified. Developmental psychopathology was initially defined by Sroufe and Rutter (1984) as *"the study of the origins and course of individual patterns of behavioral maladaptation, whatever the age of onset, whatever the causes, whatever the transformations in behavioral manifestation, and however complex the course of the developmental pattern may be."* As covered in Chapter 1, exposure to ACEs significantly increases the risk for developmental processes to go awry. The capacity to regulate emotions and related behavior is one such process that is negatively impacted when developmental adversity is part of a child's life history. When problems with emotion regulation occur (otherwise known as emotion dysregulation), this clinical presentation sets the stage for *TIP*[s] to be employed for maximum benefit. However, a foundational understanding of emotions in general needs to be established before detailed accounts of episodes or bouts of emotion dysregulation can be made.

Emotions as Response Tendencies

Although human emotions have been the subject of discussion and inquiry for more than two millennia, no consensus has ever been reached in defining what an emotion is. What has been (mostly) agreed upon is that emotions include separable components. One such component is an evaluative one in which the component serves to help us determine whether the present external experience is a relatively positive one (e.g., friends and family singing "Happy Birthday" to you at a celebration) or a negative one (e.g., a large barking dog running toward you). A second component, known as a subjective one, is closely tied to the first component in that the internal experience has a valence along the negative-positive continuum (e.g., the emotion, "happiness," feels pleasant whereas "anxiety" feels unpleasant). Emotions also possess a physiological component, including internal processes such as increased heart rate and blood pressure, sweating, muscle tension, and changes in breathing. Most of the time, this element is experienced as physiological arousal. The fourth component is a behavioral one that comprises overt motor acts governed by the gross and fine muscles of the human body. The jaw dropping open, for example, is a fine motor movement often associated with "surprise," whereas running away from a meat-eating predator is a gross motor act that is indicative of the emotion, "fear." Lastly, a cognitive component exists—various mental processes for maintaining, understanding, and using information to create knowledge and reflect—whereby people typically engage in "thinking" when experiencing emotions. For example, many of us may "think" to ourselves, "this is awesome" when being sung to by cherished loved ones for our birthday.

Given that emotions are multifaceted experiences, how can a given emotion then be understood at its most basic level? For our purposes, the notion of emotions as *response tendencies* is one simple yet elegant way to know how our emotions serve us as human beings (Gross, 1998; Gross & Barrett, 2011). Specifically, emotions are viewed as flexible response sequences elicited when an individual evaluates a situation as an important challenging one or as an opportunity (Gross, 1998). In addition to comprising the multiple components mentioned above, these tendencies can be modulated (i.e., regulated) or not, which ultimately determines the expressed emotional response, in other words, the overt emotion-related behavior (Figure 2.1).

Assessment of Emotion (Dys)Regulation

As defined in Chapter 1, emotion regulation is the capacity to adequately monitor, evaluate, and modify emotions to accomplish goals or meet the demands of the present environment (Thompson, 1994). Therefore, emotion dysregulation occurs when an individual struggles to attain their goals or engage and participate in the current moment's activity, event, or situation because their emotions weren't sufficiently attended to, assessed, or altered. For children, this outcome usually means that they weren't immersed in the activity at hand to the level of their caregivers' expectations. At the very least, the child is consequently viewed as a "failure" in the eyes of adult authority figures and perhaps

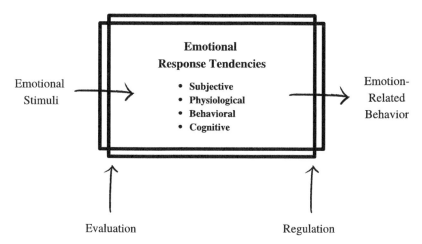

Figure 2.1 Emotions as response tendencies.

given negative verbal and/or nonverbal feedback for doing so. In the worst-case scenario, however, the child is perceived as highly impaired because the lack of participation was accompanied by dangerous behavior resulting in physical or emotional harm—an outcome referred to as *behavior dysregulation.*

Parent-completed rating scales are available to assess children's emotion regulation, including the Behavior Rating Inventory of Executive Function–Parent Report (BRIEF-PR; Gioia et al., 2002; Giola et al., 2000), Behavioral and Emotional Rating Scale, Second Edition (BERS-2; Epstein et al., 2004; Mooney et al., 2005; Sointu et al., 2014), and the Emotion Regulation Checklist (ERC; Shields & Cicchetti, 1997). The BRIEF-PR covers various domains of executive function—processes that enable people to plan, focus attention, remember instructions, and juggle multiple tasks successfully, including emotion regulation. Within the behavioral regulation scale of the questionnaire is a set of items specific to what the test developers called *emotional control* (instead of emotion regulation). The BERS-2 possesses a competency scale labeled *affective strength*, whereas the ERC assesses three emotion-specific domains—regulation, lability, and negativity. Collectively, these three measures can be used to create a comprehensive picture of a child's ability to recognize their own emotions, their emotion-related behavior, how intense their emotions are, and where they fall on the regulated-dysregulated continuum.

Another integral aspect of understanding a child's emotion regulation problems is to assess discrete episodes (or bouts or incidents) of emotion dysregulation. Such an assessment presumes that emotion dysregulation has an onset and an offset with "stuff" in between. In other words, once an episode is elicited, a set of experiences and events occurs over time that defines when a child is emotionally dysregulated until they return to a relatively regulated state. In reference to Thompson's (1994) definition of emotion regulation, both child-specific (i.e., intrinsic) and environmental (i.e., extrinsic) factors are at play when a bout of emotion dysregulation occurs. As an outcome, appropriate goal-directed activity is interfered with due to patterns of emotional experience or expression (Beauchaine, 2015; Thompson, 2019).

Four types of dysregulated emotion have been identified (Cole et al., 2017): (a) emotions that persist because of ineffective regulatory processes; (b) emotions that interfere with acceptable behavior; (c) expressed or experienced emotions that are inappropriate to the situation or circumstances; and (d) emotions that change either too quickly or not fast enough. Under-controlled/ambivalent and overcontrolled/unresponsive emotion dysregulation can occur for children exposed to developmental adversity. These deficient processes are associated with internalizing and externalizing symptoms (Kim & Cicchetti, 2010; Maughan & Cicchetti, 2002). Consequently, if a child's goal is not attained, what do they gain as a function of their dysregulation? Given what we learned in Chapter 1, the answer lies in the dichotomy between safety and threat/danger. Essentially, when a child is triggered emotionally, and that emotional experience is related to one or more memories of adversity, they consequently react and behave as if something (or someone) is threatening them, regardless of whether the threat is real or not. How this reactivity unfolds for a given child is dependent on the type(s) of adversity to which they have been exposed.

Thompson (2019) provided several examples of emotion dysregulation as a function of exposure to different types of ACEs. For instance, children who are survivors of physical abuse are particularly attuned to stimuli associated with adult anger, including anticipating anger in situations that elicit different emotions, exhibiting increased physiological vigilance when a nearby adult is angry, and showing a response bias toward facial expressions of anger (for a review, see Pollak, 2015). In contrast, children exposed to physical neglect are sensitive to signs of sadness—the emotion that people experience when a loss is perceived. In this case, the loss is all about parents being incapable of providing adequate care and limited responding to and emotional reciprocity with the child. Similarly, children growing up in a household with a mother with depression-related problems (i.e., impaired caregiver) are notably alert and attentive to their mother's emotional state. They also tend to regulate their own emotions by managing their mothers' emotions. Together, these processes increase the risk for problems with emotional development and well-being (e.g., emotion dysregulation). In all, these examples illustrate how adverse family environments combined with biological factors (e.g., altered stress neurobiology, heightened inflammation, and heritable traits) can contribute to the onset and maintenance of emotion dysregulation (Thompson, 2019).

The assessment of emotion dysregulation episodes shares similarities with assessment procedures from other behavioral healthcare fields, such as functional behavioral assessment (FBA) from the applied behavior analysis tradition (Call et al., 2017; Hadaway & Brue, 2016) and a chain analysis, which was derived within dialectical behavior therapy (Landes, 2019; Rizvi, 2019). These assessment strategies share a common cornerstone, direct observation: the information gathered comes from people who have been in close physical proximity to the child where they have directly witnessed an emotion dysregulation episode. This clinical data is typically obtained by conducting an unstructured interview. Of course, the most proximal individual to the child is the child themselves. Thus, the child is usually the first person to be interviewed. However, for various reasons, children will usually not be able to report the details of their own incident(s) of emotion dysregulation fully and accurately. A reduction in conscious awareness during the episode while in a state of heightened negative emotionality is an example of one such factor. Thus, interviewing other direct witnesses is imperative, whether those individuals include other children or adults who were present. Interviews with several individuals align with the assessment tactic of collecting information from multiple respondents as best practice, maximizing the reliability and validity of the clinical data obtained.

Steps in Identifying Emotional Dysregulation

Step One: "Get a cue." Across all three strategies, the first step is the identification of a stimulus, cue, or trigger, which generically emanates from an external source of stimulation—often a specific individual (or one or more of their features) in a child's physical presence. Operationally, the perception of a stimulus serves as the onset of an episode of emotion dysregulation. For children exposed to developmental adversity, the most salient types of stimulation are ones that come from sources of perceived threat or danger. Based on the unique history of exposure to adverse childhood experiences (ACEs), a child can also be sensitized to stimulation by sources of perceived antagonism/opposition, obstruction/thwarting, loss, and aversion, among others. These stimuli are associated with dysregulation episodes that comprise emotional experiences of anger, frustration, sadness, and disgust, respectively. Visual, auditory, olfactory, tactile, and kinesthetic stimuli can all be perceived, consequently eliciting the emotion dysregulation. In practice, something that someone says, how they say something, or how they act are the most common functional stimuli, cues, or triggers. For example, an adult caregiver's "angry voice" (regardless of the actual verbal content) can elicit a dysregulated emotional state. Also, the "sad look" on a sibling's face could serve as a stimulus leading to emotion dysregulation. Even inanimate objects reminiscent of past developmental adversity can be sources of stimulation to which a child emotionally reacts.

Step Two: "Get the feeling." The second step in assessing an emotion dysregulation episode is to ascertain all the aspects of the dysregulated emotion. These facets include evaluative, subjective, physiological, behavioral, and cognitive components as described above. The dysregulated emotion can also be one of the four types previously highlighted (Cole et al., 2017). One helpful framework to guide clinicians in identifying the dysregulated emotion and describing its various facets is the diagnostic criteria for the proposed diagnosis, Developmental Trauma Disorder (DTD), as illustrated in the Developmental Trauma Disorder Semi-Structured Interview (Ford et al., 2018). The first domain of DTD for reference is known as affective and physiological dysregulation, which includes four "symptoms":

1) inability to modulate, tolerate, or recover from extreme affect states (e.g., fear, anger, shame), including prolonged and extreme tantrums, or immobilization; this presentation typifies emotions that either persist due to ineffective regulatory processes or change either too quickly or not fast enough;
2) disturbances in regulation in bodily functions (e.g., persistent disturbances in sleeping, eating, and elimination; over-reactivity or under-reactivity to touch and sounds; disorganization during routine transitions). Although primarily physiological, this clinical picture exemplifies ineffective regulation, interference with acceptable behavior, and inappropriateness to the situation or circumstances;
3) diminished awareness/dissociation of sensations, emotions, and bodily states; this (mainly) cognitive component comprises ineffective regulatory processes, interference with acceptable behavior, or modulation that is too slow; and
4) impaired capacity to describe emotions or bodily states; as another primarily cognitive component, this clinical presentation is formally known as alexithymia.

The second domain of DTD relevant to our discussion on ascertaining the details of emotion dysregulation includes symptoms or problems that are risky, dangerous, or unacceptable. As with the first DTD domain symptoms, the dysregulated emotions can be prolonged due to ineffective regulatory processes, be inappropriate to the activity, event, or situation, and/or change either too quickly or slowly. Known as behavioral dysregulation (i.e., emotion-related behavior problems; Ford et al., 2018), examples include the following:

1) preoccupation with threat, or impaired capacity to perceive a threat, including misreading of safety and danger cues;
2) impaired capacity for self-protection, including extreme risk-taking or thrill-seeking;
3) maladaptive attempts at self-soothing (e.g., rocking and other rhythmical movements, compulsive masturbation); and
4) habitual (intentional or automatic) or reactive self-harm.

Lastly, the third DTD diagnosis domain includes symptoms and problems concerning the child themselves or other people. In other words, the child's dysregulated emotions are tied to their sense of personal identity and involvement in relationships (Ford et al., 2018). The "symptoms" below exemplify the clinical presentation of this cluster:

1) intense preoccupation with the safety of caregiver or other loved ones (including precocious caregiving) or difficulty tolerating reunion with them after separation;
2) the persistent negative sense of self, including self-loathing, helplessness, worthlessness, ineffectiveness, or defectiveness;
3) extreme and persistent distrust, defiance, or lack of reciprocal behavior in close relationships with adults or peers;
4) reactive physical or verbal aggression toward peers, caregivers, or other adults;
5) inappropriate (excessive or promiscuous) attempts to get intimate contact (including but not limited to sexual or physical intimacy) or excessive reliance on peers or adults for safety and reassurance; and
6) impaired capacity to regulate empathic arousal as evidenced by lack of empathy for, or intolerance of, expressions of distress of others, or excessive responsiveness to the distress of others.

In summary, this step in assessing an emotion dysregulation episode involves gathering information about the topographical, external, or overt behavioral manifestation of the child's emotional reaction and the intrinsic experiences that simultaneously occur. Because these internal processes aren't directly observable, identifying them is dependent on interviewing the child themselves. In contrast, others in the child's physical presence when the child was emotionally dysregulated can report on what they witnessed and observed first-hand, including the "symptoms" covered above (e.g., tantrums, body rocking, self-harm, aggression). The child can also report on the outward expressions of their dysregulation. However, if the child were to experience diminished awareness at the time of the episode, this reduced processing would likely hamper the consolidation of the episode into long-term memory, thus limiting their capacity to provide information during the interview. Therefore, whenever possible, the child should be interviewed regardless of how much they recall. Any clinical data they can provide would help better understand how their emotion dysregulation unfolds. This information is then complemented by knowledge obtained from interviews of witnesses of the episodes.

Step Three: "Get the target:" The third and final step in assessing emotion dysregulation episodes is to identify the consequences or outcomes of the child's experience; the effects on the child and their immediate environment (social and physical) must both be considered. At the very least, the primary presumption is that the dysregulation interferes with appropriate goal-directed activity, according to Beauchaine (2015) and Thompson (2019). This outlook is consistent with the World Health Organization's (2001) three-dimension definition of disability. For the first dimension, the child's emotion dysregulation is an example of **impairment** in mental functioning. Difficulties with describing emotions, self-soothing, self-protection, reading of safety and danger cues, and intimate contact exemplify the dimension of **activity limitations**. The third dimension is referred to as **participation restrictions** in typical daily activities, such as attending school, engaging in social events, and playing sports. In simple terms, the child's emotion dysregulation gets in the way of thoroughly engaging and participating in expected and developmentally appropriate activities, events, and situations. Thus, one primary goal for the third step in the interview process is to identify all the activities hampered by the child's dysregulation.

Another primary goal is to ascertain the impact of the child's emotion dysregulation on the people around them at the time of the episode and the immediate physical surroundings. For example, Cole et al. (2017) noted that dysregulation could include unacceptable or inappropriate actions, resulting in negative experiences of those individuals who were present. When mild, the exhibited behavior problems may merely lead to thoughts or ideas of others about the child that are "less than positive." In the extreme, the child can engage in aggressive behavior that endangers the physical integrity of others. Such heightened dysregulation can also be expressed in acts that are physically damaging to inanimate objects in the child's vicinity. Consequently, clinically appropriate interventions can range from teaching acceptable/appropriate behavior to intervening to decrease the risk of physical harm, respectively (covered fully in Chapter 4). Whether the child's dysregulation is associated with physical harm due to aggressive behavior toward themselves (i.e., self-injury, self-harm, or self-destruction) also needs to be determined by interviewing the child and others who may be "in the know."

Typically, assessing one episode of emotion dysregulation is not enough to accurately and comprehensively know how children experience their dysregulated emotional states and how they progress over time. For example, a given episode may have unique features that make its occurrence different than others. Such uniqueness can include the eliciting stimulus, the setting where the incident occurred, the emotion(s) experienced, the expressed behavior(s), and the outcomes of the episode. Instead, several episodes need to be assessed so that commonalities can be determined across them. When such clinical data is obtained, a pattern of emotion dysregulation often manifests. This regularity among episodes makes interventions easier to identify and conduct because the "problem" is well-known and understood in ways that make sense. In contrast, emotion dysregulation seems random and nonsensical when a pattern isn't elucidated. Clinical experience indicates that at least 3–4 episodes need to be assessed to ascertain consistency. Although identifying a pattern of emotion dysregulation is the goal, clinicians must also remember that two or more patterns are possible, which means that further clinical interviews need to be conducted to assess many more episodes.

One helpful framework to more fully understand how emotion dysregulation episodes unfold and regularities among them comes from within the treatment known as Trauma Systems Therapy (TST; Brown et al., 2014; Navalta et al., 2013; Saxe et al., 2007). Several factors are considered when assessing whether the child is experiencing emotion dysregulation. First, an episode of dysregulation is defined as changes in awareness (or consciousness), affect (or emotion), and action (or behavior) when the child is exposed to an eliciting stimulus. In TST, these indicators are known as the *3 As*. If changes do not occur across the three processes, the child is not considered to be dysregulated. Second, how often the episodes occur and to what extent they cause problems with the child's school, family, peer relationships, or themselves are determined. Third, when the child engages in risky or potentially dangerous behavior during an episode, such as aggressive or self-injurious behaviors, they are considered *behaviorally dysregulated.* From this viewpoint, the expression of emotion dysregulation is so severe that the associated behavior problems need to be distinctly labeled and targeted for intervention.

Within TST, how an episode of emotion dysregulation proceeds across time is monikered with the term, *4 Rs*, which stands for regulating, revving, re-experiencing, and reconstituting phases. Before the presence of an eliciting stimulus, the child is deemed to be emotionally *regulating* if they are actively engaged with their surroundings and effectively participating in the activity, event, or situation at hand. Once they are triggered, and an emotion dysregulation episode has begun, the earlier and milder aspects of the experience are occurring or *revving*, becoming more active or energetic. If the emotional experience becomes more intense, the child will eventually reach the phase when they feel as if they're *re-experiencing* a past incident of trauma or adversity. Lastly, before fully returning to an emotionally regulated state, the child goes through a transitional or *reconstituting* phase. The *4 Rs* is thus a simple delineation of an emotion dysregulation episode across time.

Of course, clinicians can use a standardized assessment tool to assess the effects of a child's emotion dysregulation. One such instrument is the Child and Adolescent Functional Assessment Scale (CAFAS; Hodges et al., 2000; Hodges & Kim, 2000). The CAFAS provides an objective, comprehensive assessment of a child's needs via a clinical interview. Eight life domains are covered: (a) school; (b) home; (c) community; (d) behavior toward others; (e) moods/emotions; (f) self-harm; (g) substance use; and (h) thinking. A total score and subscale scores are provided, with higher scores indicating greater impairment in day-to-day functioning. Based on substantial published research, the CAFAS is a psychometrically sound measure that demonstrates internal consistency, inter-rater reliability, and test-retest reliability

(Hodges & Gust, 1995; Hodges & Wong, 1996). Given its sensitivity to change over time (Hodges et al., 1998, 1999; Hodges & Wong, 1996), the CAFAS is a widely used treatment outcome measure. Perhaps most relevant to our discussions is that the instrument has been proven to be sensitive to improvement for children treated with parent training strategies (e.g., Parent Management Training–Oregon; Hodges et al., 2008).

Summary

To close, we now have a comprehensive assessment strategy to assess children who have been exposed to trauma and adversity. The approach detailed in this chapter takes full advantage of multi-method, multi-informant best practices in gleaning relevant clinical information. Vital knowledge to be gained in the assessment phase includes the details of the ACEs in the child's history and the current clinical presentation of the child. One cornerstone of the children's symptomatology is their emotion dysregulation. Not only can we objectively assess this regulatory process with the use of standardized questionnaires, we can also derive nuanced accounts of dysregulation episodes by conducting clinical interviews with the child and with others who were present during the incidents to "see" how the dysregulation unfolded from their eyes (and ears). We were also introduced to a framework that captures how the process is experienced over time across the *3 As* (awareness, action, and affect) and *4 Rs* (regulating, revving, re-experiencing, and reconstituting) as well as the use of standardized tools to formalize the extent of impairment associated with emotion dysregulation.

From here, we move from *assessing* to *understanding*, which we call *case conceptualization*. This therapeutic activity guides the clinician to take the gathered assessment data and turn the information into an integrated and comprehensive clinical picture of the child. From that point in the process, the creation of a treatment plan naturally and logically flows.

3

Case Conceptualization

At the end of this chapter, you will be able to:

- Define case conceptualization
- Create a clinical formulation that integrates:
  - Identified and defined primary problems
  - Predisposing, precipitating, and perpetuating factors ("3 Ps" or "Triple Ps")
    that contribute to the onset and maintenance of symptomatology
  - One or more theories of human behavior and functioning
- Identify treatment-related personal strengths, external resources, and problems

"Understand Before You Intervene"

In Chapter 2, a simple mantra was introduced to guide the work that we do as clinicians: "*Assess to understand before you intervene.*" This statement refers to the three main phases or practices that clinicians typically undergo in sequence when working with their clients or patients. The assessment phase was described in detail in the previous chapter in which clinically relevant information is collected that centers on the child's clinical presentation and symptomatology. For our purposes, the primary domains targeted for data collection comprise the often multiple and varied adversities that children can be exposed to and the consequent clinical symptoms and problems they experience. Based on what we know clinically and scientifically about children exposed to developmental adversity, a cornerstone of the child's symptomatology is their emotion dysregulation. Hence, much of the work during the assessment phase is to gather sufficient information so that the clinician is confident in knowing the child's dysregulated emotional states. Simply stated, assessment practices are conducted with the goal of clinical understanding. Without such knowledge, recommended treatments and

Trauma-Informed Parenting Program: TIP^s for Clinicians to Train Parents of Children Impacted by Trauma & Adversity, First Edition. Carryl P. Navalta.
© 2022 John Wiley & Sons, Inc. Published 2022 by John Wiley & Sons, Inc.
Companion Website: www.wiley.com/go/navalta/tipsforclinicians

therapies may be misguided and potentially harmful. Thus, before clinicians begin their interventions (in our case, parent training and education), a thorough understanding of the child's clinical picture must be ascertained; this comprehension is known as *case conceptualization.*

Case Conceptualization

At its essence, case conceptualization is the clinical understanding of a child's problems across their major psychological processes (i.e., behavioral, emotional, cognitive, and interpersonal). Although these factors are intrinsic to the child, extrinsic factors are also integral to the knowledge base for the clinician (e.g., the influence of peers on one's biopsychosocial development). Case conceptualization includes internal and external variables that result in a comprehensive picture of the child, how their problems developed, and how they can be improved. Such clinical understanding provides a "roadmap" that guides assessment, identifies targets for treatment, and highlights potential markers for clinical change. In all, case conceptualization drives every clinical activity, even when not directly stated (Winters et al., 2007).

Although based on clinical data, case conceptualization is hypothetical in that the accrued knowledge of the clinician is the "best account of the client's problems: why the client is experiencing them, what precipitates symptom onset, and why symptoms continue to occur instead of resolve." (Eells, 2015, p. 16). As a hypothesis, an initial case conceptualization can be bolstered when additional information about the child is obtained that aligns with what is currently known. On the other hand, an update may be needed if new information is misaligned with the present clinical understanding or, at its worst, a complete revision is required when sufficient data contradicts the preliminary conceptualization. Thus, case conceptualization is an evolving process that can be supported or refuted depending on what the clinician learns about the child.

The case conceptualization model presented here is primarily based on the framework outlined by Falender and Shafranske (2012). This approach to conceptualizing the child's problems is divided into two domains: (a) clinical formulation; and (b) treatment-related factors and processes. Although known by several labels (e.g., clinical case formulation, diagnostic formulation, psychotherapy case formulation), the clinical formulation is the comprehensive understanding of the nature of the child's problems. Arrival to this understanding occurs when the following information is obtained and integrated into an explainable and testable hypothesis:

1) Identified and defined primary problems
2) Predisposing, precipitating, and perpetuating factors, and
3) One or more theories of human behavior and functioning

Both clinical data and evidence from the theoretical and scientific literature are used toward developing the clinical formulation, and theory is applied to enhance the soundness of the overarching hypothesis (Falender & Shafranske, 2012).

In contrast, factors related to treatment and interventions are identified to round out and supplement the clinical formulation toward creating and formalizing the "big picture" of case conceptualization. Such variables can be divided into two types—those that "help" and those that "hinder" the therapeutic process and outcome. Helpful factors include the child's strengths and external resources or assets, whereas hindering factors are what clinicians generally refer to as problems or barriers. For example, potential resistance areas in the treatment process and the clinician's reaction to the child or family might present obstacles to progress; these hindrances may be identified ahead of time or early in treatment to allow for sufficient mitigation (Winters et al., 2007). Perhaps most importantly, the recognition of parental psychological strengths and vulnerabilities is required to maximize the impact of parent training and minimize any factors that might interfere with the caregiver-focused intervention, respectively.

In an article that this book's author and one of his former students wrote on case conceptualization (Navalta & Moore, 2016, November), we proposed that case conceptualization exists at the intersection of science and art and that the process of conceptualizing cases mirrors baking a cake. That is, precision is required in measuring and combining ingredients, heating the oven, and timing the baking: that is, the science. Master bakers, however, also draw upon their unique personality, creativity, and experience to bake a cake that transcends the ordinary; this distinctive process is the art. Likewise, a complete understanding of our clients and patients comes about by merging the science of human behavior with the artistry of the clinician. For this chapter, this baking analogy will be used as a guide for learning how to create comprehensive and accurate case conceptualizations that also possess clinical utility—a "recipe" for case conceptualization.

A Framework for Case Conceptualization

"What's the problem?"

The first step in developing a clinical formulation is identifying and defining what are known as primary problems. The term, *primary,* is used in this context because the word refers to the most critical problems to target. At first glance, the "obvious" problems that are primary would appear to be the presenting or chief complaints or the reasons for referral. However, this conclusion may not necessarily be accurate for various reasons, such as the parent minimizing or neglecting genuine problems or overblowing other ones. The child's perspective also requires consideration as they might have problematic experiences of which the parents are unaware.

In contrast, the parent might report that the child isn't performing well enough in one or more expected, typical, and developmentally appropriate activities, indicating that the child is functionally or psychosocially impaired due to their symptoms. If, for example, the parent states, *"My son isn't doing well in school."* or *"They don't have any friends.",* real problems may be at hand. What makes a problem a true primary one is based on its high level of impairment, distress, or importance (or meaningfulness or value) to the child and parents. Consequently, primary problems are targeted for intervention in the here-and-now. However, problems identified to be addressed in the future are labeled as secondary, tertiary, or other problems. In bakers' terminology, clinical symptomatology and its associated impairment, distress, and importance are the "key ingredients" of the cake itself.

Just as a baker wants the ingredients in a cake to be specific to ensure that their cake is the exact flavor they want (e.g., chocolate rather than vanilla), clinicians need to be sure that the identified problems align with the child's most salient challenges. As highlighted in Chapter 2, clinical symptoms or problems are insufficient to ascertain that the child experiences emotion dysregulation. Instead, the clinician needs to verify and document that the dysregulation interferes with daily functioning across one or more life domains. In World Health Organization terminology (2001), such interference comprises activity limitations and participation restrictions. For children negatively impacted by adverse childhood experiences (ACEs), the expression of emotion dysregulation is impairing when one or more of the following is jeopardized: (a) physical safety (e.g., self-injury or physical aggression is experienced); (b) engagement or retention in treatment; (c) home placement; (d) school functioning; and (e) healthy development (physical and psychosocial). Compromised psychosocial development includes the child's diminished ability to make and keep friends, effectively interact with peers, and function adequately within the family system. In sum, the presence of impairment is sufficient to conclude that a problem is a primary one, which necessitates immediate intervention.

Distress associated with manifest symptomatology experienced by the child as well as the importance, meaningfulness, and value of the clinical symptoms to the child or parent (or other significant adults in the child's life, such as teachers, before- and after-school staff, sports coaches, scout leaders, dance instructors, etc.) are additional characteristics that can lead the clinician to decide that the problem is a primary one and should be targeted for treatment now rather than later. Typically, distress is identified when the child verbally reports (or the parent witnesses overt expressions) that subjective experiences of discomfort or pain accompany their symptoms. For example, the child might say, *"I hate feeling that way [when I act out or shut down]."* or *"It really bothers me when I get mad at my mom and yell at her."* A parent, in contrast, might state, *"They get very upset whenever they act out."* In both cases, the present distress indicates that the problem is significant enough to be determined as primary. Relatedly, the experienced distress may contribute to the child or parent (or again, other central adults) viewing a given problem as highly important or meaningful to address through their eyes. However, many other factors can influence the extent to which a problem is perceived as critical to target for immediate intervention, such as their own subjective experience of the problem and value system. When a parent's job is on the line, for example, because they have to continually leave work to pick up their child who is dismissed early from school due to aggressive behavior, the parent would likely see that problem as a priority to address so that the chances of being fired by their employer is lessened. Collectively, distress and importance associated with a clinical problem (in addition to impairment) help the clinician identify primary problems (i.e., the ones to target first).

Before moving on to how to define primary problems, the number of problems to identify as primary at a given time needs to be briefly discussed. In short, if all problems are recognized as primary (especially when many exist), then none of them are truly priorities because they are given equal status simultaneously. Another negative consequence of identifying too many primary problems is that the therapeutic work will be insufficient due to the need to substantially divide and lessen the clinician's efforts and attention toward them. In turn, this deficiency would most likely result in ineffective treatment. To address this dilemma, a small number of primary problems should be identified (i.e., four or fewer). Targeting no more than four primary problems will allow the clinician to keep their work optimal and address multiple issues, which is often imperative for children exposed to developmental adversity.

Once the primary problems are identified, they now have to be defined. The information obtained from the assessment of emotion dysregulation episodes is used to generate definitions. As a reminder, an episode comprises the following features: (a) the eliciting stimulus, trigger, or cue; (b) the subjective, internal experience of the dysregulated emotional state; (c) the external expression of the emotion; and (d) the outcome or effects on the child and their social and physical environment. Generally speaking, problem definitions should be described in objective ways, meaning that the descriptions are empirical, fact-based, and quantitative. First, for the eliciting stimulus, this approach means that the source of stimulation should be described as part of the definition. The type of stimulus perceived should also be directly stated or indirectly implied based on the wording. Although visual and auditory stimuli are the most common elicitors, olfactory, tactile, and kinesthetic stimuli can trigger an episode. Recall from Chapter 2 that consistency exists between emotional stimuli and their corresponding elicited emotion. As a reminder, perceived sources of stimulation typically result in unique emotional states, such as the following ones:

- Threat/danger → anxiety
- Antagonism/opposition → anger
- Obstruction/thwarting → frustration
- Loss → sadness
- Aversion → disgust
- Non-acceptance → rejection
- Wrongdoing or fault → guilt
- Inadequacy, unworthiness, or dishonor → shame
- Neglect (emotional or material) → abandonment

Clinicians also need to remember that specific people in the child's presence are often sources of stimulation. Thus, a given individual could say and do things simultaneously or in quick succession that provide multiple stimuli, leading to eliciting multiple emotions. When two or more negative emotions are experienced, this co-occurring emotional state is commonly described as feeling "upset." Regardless of how many emotions are elicited, the stimulus (or stimuli) needs to be described objectively.

Second, objective definitions arise when behavioral indicators describe dysregulated emotion(s). In practice, the overt expressions or behaviors thus serve as cornerstones of definitions (i.e., emotion-related behavior). Although the child's internal experience isn't included, which makes definitions less complete, the omission leads to greater objectivity because the intrinsic aspects of the dysregulation are subjective. Motoric acts governed by the gross and fine motor muscles and the child's verbal behavior (i.e., what the child says) are the main types of behavioral indicators for inclusion in definitions of primary problems. As Kazdin (2005) noted in his parent training model, behavior is what people can see and hear in others. Examples of behavior indicative of DTD symptoms outlined in Chapter 2 include the following ones:

- Repeatedly yelling *"No, no, no!"* while stomping both feet on the ground (i.e., inability to modulate, tolerate, or recover from extreme affect states)
- Nighttime urination while asleep in bed (i.e., disturbances in regulation in bodily functions)
- Few to no words used to describe emotions (i.e., impaired capacity to describe emotions)
- Quickly walking or running into a street intersection without looking for oncoming vehicles beforehand (i.e., impaired capacity for self-protection)
- Punching their head with their own fist (i.e., habitual or reactive self-harm), and
- Hitting and kicking a younger sibling (i.e., reactive physical or verbal aggression).

When such observable behaviors, responses, or acts are incorporated, this inclusion results in definitions that are relatively non-judgmental and free of subjective appraisals, hence more reliable and valid.

Lastly, the consequences or effects of emotion dysregulation are also included in primary problem definitions. Again, outcomes include ones specific to the child. Two of which always need to be considered are from the WHO (2001) disability categorization—activity limitations and participation restrictions. These consequences, in effect, are the child not being able as expected to fully complete or participate in a given activity, event, or situation. When sufficient in magnitude (e.g., frequency, intensity, or duration), the longer-term outcomes include psychosocial or functional areas mentioned above that can be jeopardized, such as home placement, school progress, engagement and retention in treatment, and healthy development.

For example, the child's continual hitting and kicking their sibling can lead to inpatient hospital care or foster care, particularly when the aggressive behavior results in significant physical harm. A child who has ongoing bouts of yelling at their homeroom teacher while also stomping their feet will likely miss out on many in-class learning activities and thus make insufficient academic progress. The child who punches themselves in the head whenever they're told to get into the car to be driven to their counseling appointment and the parent then tells them they don't have to attend the session ends up not getting the treatment they need. Another child who urinates nightly, which interferes with sufficient sleep, will have their biobehavioral development compromised due to physical and mental fatigue. In all, these instances exemplify the types of outcomes that require inclusion in definitions of primary problems. As with stimuli and emotion-related behavior, consequences of emotion dysregulation should be described in terms that are (mostly) quantitative and based on facts to contribute to the overall objectivity of definitions.

The template below was created to help clinicians write objective primary problem definitions based on the guidelines above. The information within the parentheses is provided and written out by the clinician, which is unique to each child.

> *When (child's name) is triggered by (source of stimulation and emotional stimuli perceived), they/she/he react by engaging in (emotion-related behaviors). As a result, (child's name) experiences (activity limitations and participation restrictions). These constraints have put them/her/him at risk for (psychosocial or functional impairment [or physical harm when appropriate]).*

The main goal for the clinician is to devise definitions that are fact-based and data-driven so that objectivity is optimized, resulting in reliable and valid problems to target for intervention. These qualities will subsequently lead to creating long-term treatment goals and corresponding short-term objectives that also possess objectivity (covered in Chapter 4), which will ultimately allow the clinician (and parent) to measure progress toward them as markers of change and improvement. When the primary problems are identified and defined, the cake bread is now baked and out of the oven. The cake will have no more than four bread layers as the number of primary problems should be a maximum of four at any given time.

"The 3 Ps"

Although the bread of a cake is its most fundamental part, other components are integral to making the cake complete. One such element helps bring the bread layers together and hold them in place - the buttercream "filling" between layers. Clinically, the issue at hand is the factors contributing to the development and onset of the primary problems and the processes that maintain the children's symptomatology. These variables are *predisposing*, *precipitating*, and *perpetuating* factors (i.e., "3 Ps"). The first two *Ps* are typically referred to as risk or vulnerability factors, whereas the latter *P* is often considered an inhibitory factor (Layne et al., 2017).

This aspect of case conceptualization provides the context for primary problems. As a cake filling can vary in texture and consistency, the context is likewise largely dependent on how many and what types of relevant factors are included. In general, behavioral health problems (probably all health problems) are multifactorial, meaning that a few or many factors can play a role in their development. At its simplest, these variables can be intrinsic/internal to the child or come from somewhere in their environment (i.e., extrinsic/external processes). The biopsychosocial model (Engel, 1977, 1980) provides a valuable and robust framework to capture these factors.

In contrast to the biomedical approach that seeks to understand all phenomena at a molecular level, the biopsychosocial model takes a multi-level perspective in understanding health and health problems. Specifically, these levels include biological, psychological, and social factors and how they interact to increase the risk of developing a health problem. Biological dynamics or processes, in essence, are the physical elements of the body that are determinants of health, such as the central nervous, immune, and cardiovascular systems. Psychological factors, in contrast, include the cognitive, emotional, and behavioral systems that influence health. Given the intrinsic nature of biological and psychological processes, the model also has practical considerations in understanding the child's subjective experience as essential to health and health outcomes (Borrell-Carrió et al., 2004). On the other hand, social factors comprise various dynamics external to the child along a proximal-to-distal continuum.

The social-ecological theory of child development by Bronfenbrenner (1977, 1979) and its extension to developmental adversity by Cicchetti and colleagues (1993, 2015) as well as Belsky (1993) are most pertinent to this discussion. These developmentally grounded ecological-transactional models focus on the multiple-layered systems that impinge upon a child's maturational trajectories. The latter two models were specifically designed to capture the real-world complexities of exposure to ACEs and specify the interactions among adverse events, the developing child, and the variety of social contexts that children inhabit (e.g., family system, broader social environment, community, and culture). As proposed by Cicchetti and Lynch (1993), each level of the environment can interact with one another and with a child's constitutional and developmental vulnerabilities to predict a child's response to adversity.

The "social" domain of the biopsychosocial model is often divided between interpersonal processes and systemic or structural ones. For example, direct contacts with others and the consequences of others' actions are interpersonal dynamics that exemplify what Bronfenbrenner (1977, 1979) called the microsystem—a child's interactions with family members are a prime example. All interpersonal developmental adversity, thus, falls under this category. The term, macrosystem, is used to categorize those dynamics that comprise structural entities such as the system of care, including the school system, behavioral healthcare agencies, healthcare facilities, and child protective services departments. Also known as contextual factors (Lehman et al., 2017; Lynch & Cicchetti, 1998), overarching patterns of shared culture, norms, policies, practices, and values are also part of these dynamics. One underrecognized and minimized contextual dynamic that negatively impacts many children is systemic or structural racism—a system in which the patterns mentioned above promote racial group inequity. As implored in Chapter 2, systemic racism must be recognized as developmental adversity given the behavioral health consequences of exposure to such experiences. Relatedly, race/ethnicity is one of six domains in the Cultural Formulation Interview (Lewis-Fernández, 2016) that guides the clinician to query whether particular "background and identity" factors are germane to the individual's primary problems and subsequent treatment. The other areas covered include community belonging, language(s) spoken, country of origin, gender/sex and sexual orientation, and faith/religion.

In sum, a biopsychosociocontextual framework allows the clinician to identify and characterize the myriad factors, processes, and dynamics that can contribute to developing and maintaining primary problems. Next, we turn to the timing of these factors across development.

Bronfenbrenner (1995) used the word, *chronosystem,* to refer to the importance of historical time and developmental timing. Although he used this term in reference to the environmental events and transitions that occur throughout a child's life, the timing of biological and psychological factors also needs to be incorporated. The *3 Ps* is a simple way to capture when a given factor influences a primary problem across three periods. The first *P*, *predisposing factors*, refers to processes that typically occur more than one year before the onset of the primary problem. Predisposing factors include personal and family histories of the primary problems and biological and genetic processes. Most clinicians are aware of genetic predisposition, which refers to the genetic makeup of a child developed in utero that increases the risk of developing a health problem. In typical clinical practice, a genetic predisposition is presumed for a child when they have a biological parent or sibling with a documented or verified health problem. In rarer instances, the child has undergone genetic testing, and one or more genetic predispositions are confirmed.

Fewer clinicians, in contrast, are likely aware of what are known as epigenetic factors. Such processes are external environmental effects on genes that can influence health problems and be inherited (Simmons, 2008). For children exposed to developmental adversity, some evidence supports epigenetic modification of certain markers in various parts of the genome, particularly methylation - a mechanism for altering gene expression (Jiang et al., 2019; Lang et al., 2020). Thus, exposure to ACEs can predispose a child to develop a health problem through its effects on the genome. However, how these epigenetic changes specifically link such adversity with the development of behavioral health problems is unclear (Lang et al., 2020). What we are more certain of is that experiencing a health problem in the past predisposes a child to develop that same problem in the future, such as a depression-related primary problem increasing the risk for a later depression episode. Prior victimization and social disadvantage are also known predispositions. In all, predisposing factors are best viewed as events or processes in the distant past that contribute to the development of a primary problem.

In contrast, the latter two *Ps* are much more recent or presently occurring. Specifically, the second *P*, *precipitating factors*, comprises proximal events (i.e., within 12 months before primary problem onset) and includes recent major life stressors and adversities. For exposure to any given ACE, the experience would thus be classified as a precipitating factor if the exposure happened less than one year before the onset of a primary problem, whereas the same adversity would be labeled as a predisposing factor if its occurrence was greater than one year before the beginning of the primary problem. Because exposure to a specific type of ACE can be multiple (e.g., repeated sexual abuse across months to years), the adversity can be identified simultaneously as a predisposing and precipitating factor. Immediately post-exposure, low social support, family dysfunction, and the child's avoidance behavior are examples of precipitating factors (Trickey et al., 2012). Lastly, the third *P*, *perpetuating factors*, are those dynamics presently occurring in the child's life that maintain primary problems. One prime example that clinicians must assess for is someone in the child's social environment, such as a parent or other significant adult, who inadvertently reinforces a primary problem. As an illustration, attention-seeking disruptive behavior problems (e.g., crying, whining, and "temper" tantrums or outbursts) are perpetuated by parents whenever they attend to and react to their children's disruptions. The problems also most likely worsen if parents sometimes attend to their children when exhibiting these behaviors but ignore them at other times because they don't want to "give in" to them. In these situations, parents are, in essence, intermittently reinforcing the child's behavior problems—a type of reinforcement schedule that has been scientifically shown to strengthen or increase behavior (whether the behavior is positive/acceptable or negative/unacceptable).

In contrast to interpersonal dynamics that serve as perpetuating factors, limited or inadequate emotion regulation skills in children who experience emotion dysregulation exemplify an internal psychological process (with biological underpinnings) that can perpetuate a primary problem. Of course, training parents to teach their children emotion regulation skills is the foundation of *TIP*[s]. One final example is a parent who engages in treatment non-adherence by not bringing their child to counseling sessions due to a cultural bias against behavioral health problems or mistrust of the healthcare system.

Table 3.1 consists of a grid that juxtaposes the biopsychosociocontextual framework with the 3 Ps. Adapted from Winters et al. (2007), this chart can be used as a guide for clinicians to (a) identify as many factors as possible that contribute to the onset and maintenance of primary problems; and (b) categorize the dynamics according to their central features. Getting back to the analogy of baking a cake, we now have the recipe and ingredients of the buttercream filling, which brings together and holds the cake's bread layers in place.

"In Theory"

Another aspect that makes a cake unique and thus different from others is the flavor of the filling. Likewise, the clinical formulation of a child's primary problems becomes increasingly individualized and specific whenever the clinician can incorporate one or more theories of human behavior and functioning to help round out and complete their clinical understanding. Theories can be described as the "conceptual glue" that is useful for linking varied clinical information into a meaningful whole (Falender & Shafranske, 2012; p. 151). The application of theory typically depends on the clinician's lure to a given theory, their graduate training, the influence of supervisors' theoretical orientations, and new knowledge gained thereafter. With the ever-growing number of theories (Internal Family Systems and Critical Race Theory come to mind), the filling flavors expand, thus potentially enhancing the clinician's comprehension of the child.

Table 3.1 3 Ps across biopsychosociocontextual domains.

	Biological	Psychological	Social	Contextual/Cultural
Predisposing	• family psychiatric history • toxic exposures in utero • birth complications • developmental disorders • regulatory disturbances • genetics • inflammation • immune dysfunction • sex • neural dysfunction associated with developmental adversity	• insecure attachment • emotion dysregulation • rigid or negative cognitive style • low self-image	• exposure to ACEs • exposure to identity-based discrimination (e.g., race/ethnicity, gender, age) • late adoption • pre-adoption adversity • temperament mismatch • marital conflict	• poverty • low socioeconomic status • teenage parenthood • poor access to primary care or behavioral healthcare • structural/systemic racism
Precipitating	• serious physical problem or injury • use of alcohol or other substances • gender • inflammation • immune dysfunction • neural dysfunction associated with developmental adversity	• conflicts around identity • separation-individuation problems during developmental transitions, such as puberty onset or graduation from high school	• exposure to ACEs • family move with loss of friendships • COVID-19 pandemic-related stress	• recent immigration • loss of home • loss of a supportive service (e.g., respite services, appropriate school placement)
Perpetuating	• chronic health problem • functional impairment caused by cognitive deficits or learning disorders • endocrine dysfunction (HPA axis) • dysfunctional sleep • immune dysfunction • neural dysfunction associated with developmental adversity	• use of self-destructive coping mechanisms • help-rejecting personality style • traumatic re-enactments • emotion dysregulation	• chronic marital discord • developmentally inappropriate expectations • limited/lack of parental support	• chronically dangerous or hostile neighborhood • transgenerational problems of immigration • lack of culturally competent services • stigma about behavioral health problems and behavioral healthcare

Poznanski and McLennan (1995) devised a two-dimensional model that captures the theories of human behavior underlying each of the significant counseling and psychotherapy systems. The two poles in the model include the following (a) analytic versus experiential; and (b) objective versus subjective. The interaction of these dimensions results in four quadrants in which the theories can be mapped: (a) empiricism, (b) rationalism, (c) humanism, and (d) collectivism. Empiricism is centered on the worldview underlying science with the overarching assumption that people are separate from their environments, thus reactive and determined by those external dynamics. Human behavior is consequently a function of learning and the product of factors specific to current circumstances.

In contrast, rationalism assumes that understanding the world around us is dependent on knowing ourselves first. To that end, self-reflection is the key to greater self-understanding. Human possibility is presumed to be limited from this perspective, however, because people are not perfect. On the other hand, humanism is focused on growth-promoting subjective experience and that people are internally motivated toward development, growth, and meaningful interpersonal behavior. Problems develop when intrinsic motivation is challenged and viewed as developmental tasks with emotional undertones. Lastly, collectivism is the dominant worldview of most non-Western cultures in which growth-promoting objective experiences with others are valued. Through this lens, social processes give life meaning and purpose and people are largely dependent on interpersonal influences. As such, problems at the individual level are seen as by-products of systems-level problems. Table 3.2 outlines these four categories and the major theories within them.

Cognitive theory, in particular, has been helpful in better understanding primary problems related to trauma and adversity, especially in adults but children as well. The model hypothesizes that people with trauma-related symptomatology have a sense of ongoing threat within their environment perpetuated by negative appraisals of the adversity itself and poorly integrated or elaborated adversity memories (Ehlers & Clark, 2000). Children with exposure to ACEs have been shown to have maladaptive cognitive coping strategies (e.g., thought suppression, distraction, and rumination) and negative appraisals,

Table 3.2 Theories of human behavior across analytic-experiential and objective-subjective poles.

Empiricism	Rationalism	Humanism	Collectivism
Behavioral	Psychoanalytic	Person-centered	Systemic
Cognitive	Constructivist	Gestalt	Feminist
	Existential		

Adapted from Truscott (2010).

such as perceived alienation from others post-adversity (Ehlers et al., 2003; Stallard, 2003).

A five-factor theoretical model was developed by La Greca et al. (1996) that implicates multiple risk factors in the development of trauma-related primary problems. These processes include the following factors: (a) trauma and adversity exposure; (b) pre-existing characteristics; (c) post-adversity environment; (d) coping skills; and (e) additional stressful life events. Collectively, the model incorporates several adversity-related and environmental factors to better understand the child's symptomatology (Keller et al., 2017).

Two other theories can be considered for integration into the clinician's clinical formulation for enhanced understanding. First, maturational processes and age- and stage-dependent differences in symptomatology are cornerstones of the developmental trajectory theoretical model (Pynoos et al., 1999). This model also considers the timing of adversity exposure and how neurodevelopment and emotional development can be affected by ACEs. Other factors include proximal adversity reminders and secondary stressors, the child's social environment, and intrinsic processes. Second, the parental model (Scheeringa & Zeanah, 2001) is primarily a relational one in which parental distress is hypothesized to be a significant contributor to the child's adversity-rated primary problems. This distress is presumed to play out in parental functioning, the parent-child relationship, or familial functioning. Overprotective, reenacting, and withdrawn parenting, in particular, are predicted to perpetuate or potentiate the child's symptoms.

Although all theories reviewed above have utility regarding the clinician's development of the clinical formulation of the child, the parental model arguably is most directly applicable to *TIP^s* given its primary emphasis on targeting parenting skills and capacity. Regardless, the addition of theory improves clinical understanding by providing individualization and, hence, differentiation. In other words, each child is a unique individual, and the incorporation of theory can help clinicians capture their uniqueness. In baking terms, the theory provides "flavoring" to the buttercream and gives this section of the cake part of its distinction.

To summarize, the primary problems and their context (i.e., 3 Ps + theory) make up the clinical formulation—the "cake" bread with the flavored "filling" in between. In essence, this formulation is a well-integrated hypothesis that links the identified primary problems with predisposing, precipitating, and perpetuating factors as well as theory and provides a comprehensive explanation of the problems. As clinicians enter the intervention phase (recall the mantra, *"Assess to understand before you intervene"*), they then gather clinically relevant data that will either support their hypotheses or discredit them. In other words, the clinical formulation is testable and can be changed or updated as new information comes to light. From a baker's perspective, ingredients are typically removed or added to a recipe depending on how good the cake tastes the first time around.

Treatment-related Factors

In line with the case conceptualization framework of Falender & Shafranske (2012), this section capitalizes on processes that can impact the child's engagement in treatment and their continuation with the recommended interventions. Expanding the clinical understanding of the child to treatment-related factors thus speaks to knowing the "case" in its entirety as opposed to just focusing on the child and their primary problems. As with the 3 Ps, these factors can be either child-specific intrinsic processes or external dynamics. Simply put, the processes can help or hinder clinicians' work with their child clients. The baker knows this final part of the cake as the "frosting"—the outer covering that everyone can see (and when worthy can also taste!). Just as you would put the frosting on before a cake is ready for eating, clinicians need to identify treatment-related personal strengths, external resources/assets, and problems **before** they begin intervening. The goal of the final part of case conceptualization is to capitalize on identified strengths and resources while simultaneously minimizing problems so that treatment outcomes are maximized. This step is the last one in the case conceptualization "recipe."

Children exposed to ACEs can possess many strengths despite the adversity they've endured. The term, *survivor,* highlights the positive and growth-promoting aspects of their existence instead of being labeled as a victim, which connotes both negativity and passivity. Not only can the child have positive attributes that predate their adversity, but they can also develop strengths during and after those experiences. Various protective and promotive factors have been shown to reduce the negative consequences of exposure to trauma and adversity during childhood and adolescence (NCTSN Core Curriculum on Childhood Trauma Task Force, 2012). While protective factors buffer the effects of ACEs and their stressful aftermath, promotive factors enhance children's positive adjustment regardless of risk factors. Child-specific strengths include high self-esteem, self-efficacy, adaptive coping skills, above-average intelligence, easy temperament, and the ability to be reflective (Winters et al., 2007). Resilience, in particular, has received significant attention both clinically and scientifically as an essential characteristic related to positive outcomes—the capacity of a system to adapt successfully to challenges that threaten the function, survival, or future development of the system (Masten & Barnes, 2018).

Two other strengths that the clinician needs to assess are interrelated. First is the child's ability to establish a therapeutic relationship between them and the clinician. Such a relationship is considered the number one factor associated with positive outcomes regardless of treatments provided. The child's "likability" and interpersonal skills, especially with adults, are two attributes that can help them form good working relations with the clinician. Prior positive experiences with former clinicians and success in previous treatment are related child strengths. Second is the child's capacity to collaborate with the clinician in working toward specific goals and objectives. This collaboration between the child and clinician is known as the therapeutic or treatment alliance. Because the treatment goals cannot be achieved without this alliance, assessment of the working partnership is critical in the overall conceptualization of the case (Falender & Shafranske, 2012). For the alliance to develop, the child must have the ability to agree with the clinician on the primary problems to be targeted (and corresponding treatment goals) and the capacity to agree on the treatments and interventions to work on those problems toward goal attainment. In all, every strength that the child can "bring to the table" for use in treatment needs to be ascertained.

To complement the child's strengths, external dynamics in the form of resources and assets also require identification. In reference to the biopsychosociocontextual framework, both interpersonal and systemic processes can be called upon advantageously to facilitate and support the child's treatment. Of course, the most important person in the child's life is typically their parent(s). However, other significant adults in the child's social sphere should also be identified. Such potential individuals include extended family members (e.g., grandparents, aunts, uncles), schoolteachers, before- and after-school staff, sports coaches, scouts leaders, and performance and creative arts instructors. Possible assets at the systems level comprise the child's social support network, the school at large, and community-based organizations, such as churches and town- and nonprofit-based youth centers (e.g., YMCA). Returning to the notion of resilience, a stable and committed parent, caregiver, or other adult is the single most common factor for children to develop this characteristic, although other sociocontextual systems contribute to its development (Masten & Barnes, 2018). The African proverb, "It takes a village to raise a child.", is correct, and perhaps even more so when the child at stake is one with behavioral health problems associated with a history of exposure to developmental adversity.

Lastly, a case conceptualization isn't complete without considering treatment-related problems. Identifying these problems beforehand will allow the clinician to address the issues as soon as possible and thus increase the chances that the beginning of treatment will be a positive experience. This early identification will hopefully also help to prevent the occurrence of future problems. Commonly known as barriers, these factors can either emanate from within the child or be external to them from somewhere in their ecosystem. One problem that must always be determined is the child's internal motivation for change and participation in treatment. Clinical experience has demonstrated that the clinician is not the primary source of the (child) client's progress, improvement, and success in treatment, but rather is a facilitator of change that occurs as a direct function of the work and effort of the client. In other words, progress is based on how diligently the client works in treatment; success is hampered if the child's motivation to put in the effort is limited. In parallel, because the child is dependent on their parent to receive treatment (e.g., informed consent, payment for services, transportation to/from treatment sessions), low internal motivation on the parent's part will consequently lead to the child experiencing less engagement and retention in treatment.

Relatedly, if the child believes that they don't have a behavioral health problem or that the problem *"isn't really that bad,"* they are likely in the stage of change model (Prochaska & DiClemente, 1983) known as *precontemplation* (i.e., no problem is acknowledged and thus no intention nor plan to change exists), or the *contemplation* stage (in which the child considers the possibility that they have a problem but are not committed to change). In contrast, the child may believe that any apparent problem is not their fault or responsibility; instead, they believe that someone else is the causal factor. Other treatment-related cognitive problems include limited insight and relatively low intelligence. In all, several different cognitive processes may be present that can serve as barriers to the child participating in treatment.

A variety of systems barriers (i.e., environmental, familial, interpersonal, contextual) can be present that can interfere with treatment as well. For one, if no reliable and consistent transportation is available to the child (and parent), then the child is consequently restricted from engaging in treatment. Scheduling treatment sessions among the child, parent, and clinician may also be quite challenging based on how busy everyone is and whether their schedules align to hold sessions. If the child has younger siblings who are dependent on their parent's care, the absence of or limited access to childcare may be another factor that would result in the child's lowered participation in treatment. As highlighted in the Cultural Formulation Interview (American Psychiatric Association, 2013), issues related to languages spoken and the country of origin of the child and family might influence the primary problems and the recommended treatments to address them. Difficulty in understanding each other would make developing a treatment alliance between the child and clinician challenging. Also, the provision and reception of treatment itself would be compromised if a language barrier were present between them. Likewise, differences in identity and background between the child and clinician could also lead to a misunderstanding that could, in turn, disrupt the treatment alliance and interventions. If parents are to be directly involved in treatment, a variety of limitations on their part may be present that could hamper engagement, such as relatively low intelligence, limited insight, and shortcomings in psychological mindedness. Stigma related to behavioral healthcare could also be experienced by the child or parent that could interfere with their treatment participation. Lastly, the involvement of child protective services with the child and their family may be an anxiety-provoking circumstance associated with avoidance of any treatment.

In these examples, the child's potential to begin and stay in treatment is compromised. Therefore, clinicians must consider these issues and address the problems as soon as possible so that the child can optimally benefit from treatment. If the problems aren't adequately resolved in a timely manner, treatment may be curtailed, fail, or not begin at all. Together with identifying the child's strengths and available external assets, knowing treatment-related problems is the "frosting" that completes the cake. Understanding these factors rounds out the clinician's case conceptualization. The identified strengths and resources can be used to facilitate and support the child's treatment, and problems can be addressed before or soon after treatment begins to lessen their interference with interventions.

An accurate and comprehensive case conceptualization requires a significant amount of data gathering. Chapter 2 delineates the various ways that such information can be collected, including clinical interviews with the child, parent, and collateral contacts; use of rating scales and other questionnaires; direct observation of the child; self-monitoring; and review of clinical records. In addition, the Case Conceptualization Development Form can be used to document and organize the gathered data and referenced to devise the case conceptualization (see Appendix A).

Final "Food for Thought"

Within the practice of behavioral healthcare, case conceptualization and treatment planning (covered in Chapter 4) need to be built upon a science-based foundation so that primary problems are treated quickly and effectively. This process requires identifying and defining (a) no more than four primary problems; (b) the 3 Ps that contribute to them, together with a theoretical framework to provide the "glue"; and (c) treatment-related personal strengths, external resources, and problems. Compiling, assessing, and utilizing data in our conceptualizations and resulting treatment plans can be viewed as the efficient "science" of the work. Clinicians also need to balance this process with altering interventions when the child's primary problems aren't sufficiently improving. The clinician must generate revised formulations, and corresponding treatment approaches as needed, often during any given moment of the therapeutic journey. Such revisions require flexibility, creativity, and even the ability to shift conceptual lenses; these facets make up the "art" of baking a cake, in other words, developing the final case conceptualization.

4

Treatment Planning

At the end of this chapter, you will be able to:

- Articulate the four main components of a comprehensive and effective treatment plan
- Create a plan undergoing the four elemental processes:
  1) Developing goals
  2) Constructing objectives
  3) Creating interventions
  4) Determining diagnoses
- Explain the common facets across the science-based treatments
- Know when to refer for a psychiatric medication evaluation
- Discuss effective pharmacological interventions for adversity-related symptoms

Chapter 3 highlighted the middle phase of our guiding mantra, *"Assess to understand before you intervene"*, which is the clinical understanding of the child known as case conceptualization. Following the case conceptualization is developing the treatment plan by establishing the interventions to be provided, which is the third phase of our mantra. As we now know, the cornerstone of case conceptualization is the identification and definition of primary problems—the targets of our recommended treatment at present based on their significant impairment, distress, and importance to the child and parent. In parallel, treatment planning is anchored by the long-term goals—the endpoints or destination of the "therapeutic road." However, to arrive at these goals, markers along the way are needed to determine that the child is on the "right road." These indicators, known as short-term objectives, are used to determine whether progress is being made (i.e., the child is improving). Treatments and the specific interventions within them can then be created

Trauma-Informed Parenting Program: TIPs for Clinicians to Train Parents of Children Impacted by Trauma & Adversity, First Edition. Carryl P. Navalta.
© 2022 John Wiley & Sons, Inc. Published 2022 by John Wiley & Sons, Inc.
Companion Website: www.wiley.com/go/navalta/tipsforclinicians

once the goals and objectives are articulated. Lastly, clinically appropriate diagnoses can be determined when called for, such as when health insurance companies require them for payment of behavioral healthcare services. At times, further treatment is needed beyond the scope of the clinician. Such circumstances are especially true when the child's clinical picture indicates that the child may benefit from psychopharmacological means. Thus, the clinician must understand the psychiatric evaluation and medications that are helpful for adversity-related symptoms.

In short, treatment planning is a process that outlines and describes the recommended course of treatment. Erk (2008) provided the following key clinical questions to answer as instrumental to the practice:

- Do you know which problems will be targeted in the treatment plan?
- Have measurable goals been generated?
- Has the level of care been determined?
- Has a treatment modality been selected?
- Do you know which treatment works best for the target problem?
- Have treatments been matched to the client's level of change?
- Have treatments been matched to what the client is ready to do?
- Are the treatments sensitive to salient client characteristics?

Developing the Treatment Plan

The treatment planning protocol outlined in this chapter is based on Jongsma et al. (2014), although updated and adapted for children with symptoms associated with exposure to adverse childhood experiences (ACEs). As these authors noted, an accurate and comprehensive assessment of the child allows for the formulation and implementation of the treatment plan. However, Chapter 3 (and our guiding mantra) illustrates how case conceptualization is also a vital precursor to planning for treatment. For treatment plans to have clinical utility and be effective, they must include three core components (Jongsma et al., 2014). First, the plan should be specific, not global. That is, sufficient information needs to be included in the plan that details the particulars of the treatments and interventions, including the targeted problems and treatment modalities. Second, the plan needs to be individualized rather than generalized. Instead of a "cookie-cutter" approach to treatment planning, a personalized plan considers the child's unique strengths and needs. Lastly, the plan should include measurable goals and objectives so that progress and improvement in the child can be reliably and validly assessed and documented.

Typically, the first step in treatment planning is to identify the problems to be targeted. The problems can be labeled as primary (i.e., intervene now), secondary (intervene later), or other (much later or perhaps sooner, depending on progress made with the former problems). As discussed in Chapter 3, no more than four problems should be targeted at one time. This restriction to a small number of primary problems usually results in therapeutic work that is more efficient and consequently more effective. Another factor that should be included in problem identification is that the problems should closely match the child's needs and priorities (Jongsma et al., 2014). As a reminder, the child's needs are ascertained by the presence of significant psychosocial/functional impairment and distress. Such a situation is evident when the child's symptoms interfere with their participation in expected, developmentally appropriate activities and events. In parallel, priorities are identified when the child or parent indicates that clinical problems have great importance, meaningfulness, or value to them. Together, the clinician uses these essential attributes to identify up to four primary problems to target at present. As these problems are resolved, others can be added to the problem list.

The second step in creating the treatment plan is defining the primary problems. As stated above, treatment plans require specificity in that enough information is included for clarity of understanding. This characteristic is especially needed for definitions of the primary problems. When adequate details are included in definitions, the problems are clearly evident for the child, parent, clinician, and anyone involved in their treatment. Such transparency is also maximized when definitions are operationally based (i.e., inclusive of procedures, actions, or processes). Consequently, primary problems can be observed and assessed when their definitions possess both specificity and operationalization.

Chapter 3 provides the following template for defining a primary problem that centers on the child's emotion dysregulation:

> When (child's name) is triggered by (source of stimulation and emotional stimuli perceived), they/she/he react by engaging in (emotion-related behaviors). As a result, (child's name) experiences (activity limitations and participation restrictions). These constraints have put them/her/him at risk for (psychosocial or functional impairment [or physical harm when appropriate]).

In analyzing the components of the definition within this template, several key features are evident. First, a stimulus, cue, or trigger is identified that elicits the problem in question. Second, behaviors expressed or exhibited as integral to the child's emotion dysregulation are included. Behavior is typically incorporated in operational definitions, such as this one, because of its ability to be directly witnessed by people in the individual's vicinity (i.e., seen or heard by others). Third, activities that the child is expected to participate in, but is challenged to do so because of their dysregulation, are also part of the definition. Fourth, areas of the child's life that are negatively impacted by their decreased participation (e.g., family, school, social) are also contained. These aspects of the definition collectively allow for episodes of emotion dysregulation to be observed and measured. In line with the recommendation that problems identified in the treatment plan should closely follow the diagnostic criteria used for reference (Jongsma et al., 2014), this definitional template is also consistent with the proposed diagnosis, *Developmental Trauma Disorder* (DTD; Ford et al., 2018).

The clinician should recall from the previous chapter that the primary problems are identified and defined when developing their case conceptualization. Therefore, the first two steps highlighted above don't need to be taken. Instead, the clinician can copy the primary problems and place them on the treatment plan. If only life could always be that simple . . . .

The next step of treatment planning involves the delineation of long-term treatment goals. In short, one overarching goal is identified for each primary problem. Although goals seem straightforward at first glance, clinicians typically outline and describe therapeutic activities toward goal attainment instead and may or may not include the actual goals. For example, the following "goal" highlights this issue:

> The child will participate in weekly individual counseling and learn three new coping skills.

This definition describes that a type of intervention (i.e., counseling) will be provided as well as the modality (i.e., individual versus group) and frequency (i.e., weekly) of the work. In addition, the description includes a process that will occur (i.e., learning) and a resulting skillset (i.e., coping). However, a decrease in symptomatology and impairment is implied and not stated. Improved psychosocial functioning is also not articulated. Together, such a definition is misleading as actual progress and improvement markers are missing.

In contrast, a more valuable and productive way to define treatment goals is to focus on the fact that they are outputs, endpoints, or outcomes. Goals are, in other words, the destination of the therapeutic journey or road to improved functioning. To comprise this perspective in identifying and defining goals, the clinician merely has to write the converse or opposite of the primary problem and begin the definition with this phrase: *At the end of treatment*. Therefore, the template for writing treatment goals is as follows (again, the clinician fills in the information within the parentheses):

> At the end of treatment, when (child's name) is triggered by (source of stimulation and emotional stimuli perceived), they/she/he react by engaging less in (emotion-related behaviors). As a result, (child's name) experiences greater participation in (activities, events, or situations). This increased engagement puts them/her/him at higher chances for (psychosocial or functional improvement).

As defined, the treatment goal is simply that the child experiences fewer expressions of emotion dysregulation when triggered, is less challenged with participating in expected activities, and consequently is less impaired. In other words, *"Problem solved!"*

For the next step in treatment planning, long-term goals are broken down into short-term objectives. Because goals are the culmination of the work, objectives are milestones as the child moves forward to the end of treatment. However, the duration of an episode of care is usually not predictable in real-world practice. Even when a manualized treatment is used with a fixed number of sessions, the actual provision of interventions and clinical gains made are almost always longer than the "prescribed" treatment as written. Regardless of how long treatment truly is, the clinician can still demarcate points in time after treatment begins to reference how much the child has made progress and improved. This approach to constructing objectives is easily effected by starting the definition with the phrase, *"After (# weeks/months) of treatment,"* in which the clinician provides the information within the parentheses. In this approach, the clinician chooses timeframes to monitor and assess the child's progress relative to the beginning of treatment. The onset of the therapeutic work thus provides the anchor in time.

An example to illustrate this approach is a manualized treatment that includes 12 sessions to be conducted weekly. Consequently, the work is expected to last three months when the long-term goals are expected to be attained. Because the clinician decides ahead of time that behavior change should be noticeable every three weeks or so, they choose to define four objectives and write them (at least the introductory phrases) as follows:

> Objective #1: *"After three weeks of treatment...."*
> Objective #2: *"After six weeks of treatment...."*
> Objective #3: *"After nine weeks of treatment...."*
> Objective #4: *"After twelve weeks of treatment...."*

Of course, the clinician has leeway in choosing what timeframes to use, typically based on their clinical knowledge, experience, and expertise (or pre-determined by the agency for which they work). A different clinician using the same manual may, in contrast, decide that three objectives make better clinical sense and operationalize them in monthly intervals (i.e., one month, two months, and three months after treatment begins). Irrespective of the interval chosen, objectives are established so that the child can attain them in a series of steps. The clinician determines the total number of steps, which is relatively independent of total treatment duration given that the clinician usually does not know the length ahead of time. When combined, the sequential achievement of all objectives leads to accomplishing the treatment goal.

As with the definition of treatment goals, objectives are best understood as the converse or opposite of primary problems. They also have the most utility when defined operationally and with specificity. Fundamentally, objectives are short-term, behaviorally measurable sub-goals as steps toward the overarching treatment goal (Jongsma et al., 2014). Returning to the definition template for defining goals, the clinician can see that one significant aspect of the definition is *"engaging less in emotion-related behaviors."* Consequently, the clinician has the option to define a short-term objective by a decrease in these behaviors in one or more of their operationally defined characteristics. These facets are typically a given behavior's frequency, duration, and intensity/magnitude. Second, the goal definition includes *"fewer activity limitations and participation restrictions."* Conversely, participation can be defined by its frequency and duration. When combined, the complete template for defining a short-term objective is as follows:

> After (# weeks/months) of treatment, when (child's name) is triggered by (source of stimulation and emotional stimuli perceived), they/she/he react by engaging less (frequency, duration, and/or intensity) in (emotion-related behaviors). As a result, (child's name) experiences greater participation (frequency, duration) in (activities, events, or situations).

Once short-term objectives are established, the following step is to identify and prescribe interventions. For clinicians who provide counseling and psychotherapy, interventions include therapeutic practices, techniques, and tools used to help the child and facilitate their work in achieving the defined objectives (Jongsma et al., 2014). Generally, at least one intervention is recommended to address each objective. The clinician may also decide that a psychiatric medication evaluation is warranted, which is described later in this chapter. New interventions are added to target the shortcomings if objectives are not achieved with sufficient work or are only partly met. At the very least, prescribed interventions are based on the child's symptomatology and clinical needs and the clinician's skill set, experience, and expertise.

Most importantly, scientific advances in the field of developmental adversity indicate that several treatments are effective in addressing symptoms and problems associated with exposure to ACEs. The research evidence also points to common clinical practices across these interventions. Thus, the clinician should strongly consider a science-based approach to treatment planning, which is also seen as "best practice." A review of these treatments and practices is provided below.

Scientifically Validated Treatments and Practices

The recent, extensive reviews by Dorsey et al. (2017) and Jensen et al. (2020) highlight cognitive behavior therapy with a specific focus on trauma-related symptomatology (CBT-T) as having the most substantial scientific support for the treatment of clinical symptoms and problems of children exposed to ACEs. Notably, the evidence also indicates that CBT-T can be effective when provided in different modalities, including individual counseling and psychotherapy (child), child + caregiver, and group work (child). In addition, eye movement desensitization and reprocessing therapy is strongly recommended for 1st-line treatment, with parent-child relationship enhancement and group psychoeducation as 2nd-line treatments as some empirical evidence exists for their efficacies.

CBT as a general treatment model centers on targeting cognitions (thoughts), emotions (feelings), and behaviors (actions) of individuals who are experiencing behavioral health problems. Underlying the treatment is the presumption that these three processes are interconnected and have reciprocal influences on each other. Consequently, intervening at the level of thoughts, feelings, and behavior is predicted by the model to result in progress and improvement. CBT-T possesses its uniqueness by integrating one or more cognitive theories of trauma- and adversity-related symptomatology. As described in Chapter 3, cognitive theory hypothesizes that people with clinical symptoms and problems have a sense of ongoing threat within their environment; this experience is perpetuated by (a) negative appraisals of the adversity itself; and (b) poorly integrated or elaborated memories of exposure to trauma and adversity (Ehlers & Clark, 2000). Children exposed to developmental adversity can have, for example, maladaptive cognitive coping strategies and negative appraisals. Not surprisingly, cognitive processing was identified by Dorsey et al. (2017) as one of six practice elements found in the CBT-T family of treatments and provided in combination with one or more of the others. These additional components include psychoeducation about trauma prevalence, impact, and intervention, emotion regulation training, imaginal exposure, *in vivo* exposure, and problem-solving. Similarly, the common elements found by Jensen et al. (2020) in most of the recommended models are psychoeducation, coping skills, exposure, cognitive restructuring, and parenting support and skills.

Psychoeducation is an intervention focused on transferring knowledge of a health problem and its treatment to allow individuals to cope with the problem, increase their treatment adherence, and experience greater treatment effectiveness (Ekhtiari et al., 2017). Psychoeducation typically includes providing information specific to a given health problem and more general information, such as promoting a healthy lifestyle and identifying life stressors (Motlova et al., 2017). Delivering information to family members on living with a health problem by integrating emotional and motivational factors is also conducted to increase their understanding of the problem's effects and help the individual as well as clinicians (Ekhtiari et al., 2017; Motlova et al., 2017). Specific to children with histories of exposure to ACEs and their families, such information covers post-traumatic stress symptoms, other symptoms and problems associated with exposure to trauma and adversity, the prevalence of trauma exposure, and recovery and treatment. Another vital area to review is how the social environment can help or hinder the child's psychosocial functioning. Besides the child learning to connect their symptoms with their exposure to developmental adversity, the overall goal of psychoeducation is to increase the child's and parents' understanding of reactions to trauma and adversity and the likelihood that they will collaborate with the clinician in treatment. Relevant handouts or information sheets can be used to complement verbal communication by clinicians—many of which can be found on the website of the National Child Traumatic Stress Network. As cogently described by Jensen et al. (2020), psychoeducation is essentially to *"explain, validate, and normalize"* (p. 392).

Coping refers to how people detect, appraise, deal with, and learn from stressful experiences; it comprises skills, strategies, and processes vital to adaptation and survival (Zimmer-Gembeck & Skinner, 2016). In Jensen et al.'s (2020) review of science-based treatments, the authors identified several coping skills taught across the models to address a child's dysregulation, such as relaxation, controlled breathing, emotion identification and monitoring, cognitive coping, distraction, and mindfulness. With an enhanced ability to cope and regulate themselves through treatment, the child consequently develops a decreased tendency to engage in avoidance behavior elicited by either adversity-related stimuli or daily stressors and experience episodes of emotion dysregulation. Jensen et al. (2020) also correctly pointed out that teaching coping skills in one setting (e.g., outpatient clinic) does not necessarily generalize to other settings, such as the real-life world of the child. One substantial benefit of *TIP^s* that addresses this shortcoming is that the parent is the one who teaches their child to improve their capacity to regulate emotions and related behavior in the "real world," in particular within their home setting. In other words, the parent is the teacher in this instance, not the clinician. Parent training models, in general, are successful in large part due to their focus on teaching skills at the point of need by someone vital to the child's health and well-being (i.e., parents or other caregivers). Regardless of the modality, teaching coping skills (including emotion regulation skills) is instrumental to a science-based approach to treatment and thus should be a vital part of the conversation in treatment planning.

Exposure and cognitive restructuring are cornerstones of many forms of cognitive behavior therapy for children, adolescents, and adults. For example, these interventions are the two most common practice elements in science-based treatments for child and adolescent anxiety problems (Higa-McMillan et al., 2016). Exposure is a process by which the individual intentionally and proactively "exposes" themselves to an emotional stimulus such that an emotion is elicited. The person then can learn how to cope with or regulate the experienced emotion and accompanying arousal in real time. With a sufficient number of exposures, coping and regulation improve with practice, and the magnitude of the emotion decreases as well.

In contrast, cognitive restructuring focuses on cognitive processes (i.e., thoughts, beliefs, ideas, attributions) as the targets of therapeutic change. The presumption is that symptomatology includes various cognitions that are erroneous, irrational/illogical, distorted, unduly negative, and the like. When cognitions are restructured with treatment so that they are more accurate, logical, straightforward, and less negative/more positive, this change is posited to have therapeutic benefits for the individual's emotions and behaviors.

For children exposed to ACEs, their adversity-related emotions, memories, and cognitions are the targets of treatment. With exposure tasks, both emotions and memories of the adverse experiences are typically elicited. This process allows the child to confront both the stimuli that serve as reminders of the trauma and adversity as well as memories of the experiences themselves (often labeled by the child as being "bad," "awful," or "scary"). As described by Jensen et al. (2020), the child learns via exposure *"to master trauma avoidance, fear, and other negative trauma-related symptoms"* (p. 393). Exposure work mainly involves imaginal and *in vivo* techniques (Keller et al., 2017). Although imaginal exposure historically involved describing and retelling the adversity memory in treatment sessions with the clinician, newer exposure techniques include trauma and adversity narration in different forms. For example, a child participating in EMDR therapy is tasked with internally remembering their worst experience without verbal descriptions or recordings (Barron et al., 2019; Manzoni et al., 2021), whereas drawing and writing about the memory are options in the CBT-T treatment, Cognitive Behavioral Intervention for Trauma in Schools (Jaycox, 2004).

In contrast, *in vivo* (or live) exposure demands that the child confront activities, events, and situations that they typically avoid because of the adversity memories and feeling of danger that are elicited. To concisely capture the heart of exposure work regardless of its manner of execution, the author of this manual introduced the phrase, *"Confront to conquer."* In all, exposure tasks complement therapeutic activities targeting cognitions.

Cognitive restructuring for children negatively impacted by exposure to ACEs centers primarily on the types of cognitive processes outlined by Ehlers and Clark (2000). As a reminder, these cognitions include negative appraisals of the adverse experiences, poorly integrated or elaborated adversity memories, and maladaptive cognitive coping strategies. Thus, cognitive work involves identifying and correcting these maladaptive cognitions, reducing the child's symptoms and problems. For example, Cognitive Therapy for post-traumatic stress disorder (PTSD; Smith, 2010) features therapeutic activities for the child to elaborate on and develop trauma and adversity memories into clear descriptions. The treatment also helps the child identify negative appraisals of the adversity and its effects, and decrease the use of unhelpful cognitive coping strategies. Although cognitive work combined with exposure is integral to the child's treatment, targeting parents is also critical. Such interventions acknowledge the importance of extrinsic factors in the child's behavioral health, particularly the family system.

Most science-based treatments for children exposed to ACEs with behavioral health problems have components geared toward parents (Jensen et al., 2020; Keller et al., 2017). Especially for younger children, parents and other caregivers can help the child in the therapeutic process and provide crucial information to the clinician in better understanding the child's development in general and their clinical symptoms and problems in particular. Relevant goals for parenting work include the following: (a) a greater understanding of the child's trauma and adversity experiences; (b) increased emotional support for the child; and (c) processed emotions and cognitions as well as overall reduced negativity associated with the child's exposure to ACEs (e.g., guilt or the belief that they are primarily responsible for their child's problems; Jensen et al., 2020; Keller et al., 2017). As the individual with the most control of the child's access to privileges and desired tangibles, the parent can also be instrumental in the treatment process by reinforcing or incentivizing the child to practice skills introduced in treatment between sessions. In addition, parent-focused interventions can improve parenting practices, which can be especially needed when the child has disruptive behavior problems. Such a change in the parent can also have the added benefit of them developing a sense of agency and enhanced effectiveness in their parenting role, as well as decreased parent-related stress.

A prototypical example of parenting work is Trauma-Focused Cognitive-Behavioral Therapy (TF-CBT; Brown et al., 2020). In the intervention component, Parenting Skills, the parent learns about traumatic behavioral responses and possible connections to the child's behavioral problems. This work also helps the parent recognize potential trauma reminders (known as antecedents within TF-CBT) to these behaviors and possible consequences, such as inadvertently reinforcing the behavior problems by socially attending to them. The clinician also provides education about effective parenting skills and teaches the parent these strategies. When clinically indicated, the clinician collaborates with the child and parent to develop an individualized behavior intervention plan. In "conjoint child-caregiver sessions," the child is tasked to share the trauma narrative with the caregiver. The clinician also encourages joint positive communication between the child and caregiver about the narrative. Lastly, work is conducted to engage the parent and child in safety planning and discussions about terminating treatment. Collectively, caregiver-directed interventions within TF-CBT are conducted so that parents can positively influence traumatic impact and children's treatment outcomes (Brown et al., 2020).

At this point, the reader might be wondering how *TIP^s* fits in with the four practice elements described above that are found in the science-based treatments. At first glance, the parenting support and skills component is an obvious choice for *TIP^s* to be categorized, given that the treatment is fundamentally a parent training intervention. Although that identification is valid, recall that the therapeutic target of *TIP*^{s} is the child's emotion dysregulation. This emphasis on a specific regulatory process is distinct from focusing on the child's "behavior problems." Rather than teaching parenting skills and developing a plan with the overall goal to decrease the problems, *TIP*^{s} specifically facilitates the parent's capacity to help their child better regulate their emotions and related behavior when they are triggered by adversity-related stimuli. As such, the treatment is best viewed as an integration of the second practice element identified by Jensen et al. (2020), namely coping skills (and precisely emotion regulation skills), and the parenting support and skills element. Although some psychoeducation is provided in *TIP*^{s}, the treatment leaves exposure and cognitive restructuring as future therapeutic work of the clinician with the child. *TIP*^{s} may be provided, however, in conjunction with pharmacotherapy or psychopharmacological treatment.

In some instances, the child experiences symptomatology that is substantially impairing or distressing, which clinically indicates a pharmacotherapy referral. When the child exhibits one or more of the following symptoms and problems, such a referral is generally warranted (Wilens & Hammerness, 2016):

- Self-harm or suicidality
- Threats of dangerous harm to others
- Severe or anger-related outbursts
- Auditory or visual hallucinations
- Marked withdrawal or isolation
- Weight loss with no medical cause
- Severe substance abuse
- Binging and/or purging

The prescribing clinician usually conducts a comprehensive evaluation to help determine whether a psychiatric medication trial is recommended. This assessment should include obtaining information provided by the parent and interviewing the child, especially when they are relatively younger and thus less able to verbally communicate reliable and thorough information. A complete evaluation comprises these domains and clinical activities:

- Psychiatric history
- Medication history
- Medical, developmental, social, & school history
- Family history
- Mental status examination
- Diagnosis
- Treatment plan

To date, insufficient scientific evidence exists to recommend specific medications. In the Practice Parameter for the assessment and treatment of children and adolescents with trauma-related symptoms (Cohen et al., 2010), selective serotonin reuptake inhibitors (SSRIs) are identified for "consideration." These medications include citalopram, fluoxetine, and sertraline. The Parameter also identified the following medications as possibly helpful: α- and β-adrenergic blocking agents, novel antipsychotic agents, non-SSRI antidepressants, mood-stabilizing agents, and opiates. More recently, Jensen et al. (2020) concluded that no medications are recommended based on the science to date to treat trauma-related symptoms in children. Instead, psychopharmacology should be considered when co-occurring conditions are present that have been scientifically shown to respond to pharmacological agents (e.g., depression, anxiety, and attention problems) or to target specific symptoms that are carefully and consistently tracked, which is consistent with the recommendations of Wilens and Hammerness (2016).

Because the clinician usually interacts and communicates with the child and parent more frequently than the prescriber, they are in a prime position to monitor and assess whether a prescribed medication is helpful or not. More specifically, the clinician can ascertain a beneficial outcome or anticipated positive effect for which a medication is prescribed when they assess for changes in symptoms and problems. Such improvement can include, for example, better mood (if a depression problem is present), fewer physical complaints (when anxiety is problematic), and less distractibility (when a medication is prescribed for an attention problem). The clinician can also track possible side effects or adverse reactions. These experiences can be either mild (e.g., low intensity and infrequent headaches), moderate (e.g., significant change in appetite and body weight, bothersome and frequent initial insomnia), or severe (e.g., intense, life-threatening aggression; Wilens & Hammerness, 2016).

In summary, the clinician has at their disposal several scientifically supported treatments to choose from when creating a treatment plan. Strongly recommended ones include cognitive behavior therapy with a specific focus on trauma-related symptomatology (CBT-T) and eye movement desensitization and reprocessing therapy (Jensen et al., 2020). As a treatment "family," CBT-T possesses the added benefit of providing the treatment in different modalities, namely individual child, child + caregiver, and group counseling and psychotherapy with multiple children. Moreover, these treatments have several practice elements that the clinician can decide to provide to address a given short-term objective. The core components are (a) psychoeducation; (b) coping skills; (c) exposure and cognitive restructuring; and (d) parenting support and skills. When warranted, the clinician can refer the child for psychopharmacological treatment. Such a referral would be clinically indicated if the child experiences specific symptoms or symptom clusters that have been scientifically validated to respond to psychiatric medications. Thus, treatment plans for children with behavioral health problems associated with exposure to developmental adversity can be developed with precision, personalization, and scientific backing.

Diagnosis

The final step in treatment planning is determining and making a diagnosis. Although not necessarily required in some settings (e.g., school-based counseling), a valid diagnosis can be associated with creating an effective treatment plan. Diagnoses should be based on assessing the child's present symptomatology, which comprises behavioral, cognitive, emotional, and interpersonal symptoms and their related impairment or distress. At the very least, a diagnosis can help the clinician identify primary problems. In fact, primary problems more often than not align with either an overarching diagnosis (e.g., Post-Traumatic Stress Disorder [PTSD], Major Depressive Disorder, Social Anxiety Disorder) or a symptom cluster/domain within a given diagnosis, such as the "inattention" cluster within the diagnosis of Attention Deficit Hyperactivity Disorder. The clinician should first consider one of the trauma- and stressor-related disorders in DSM-5 (American Psychiatric Association, 2013a). These diagnoses are relevant because they are predicated on the child being exposed to trauma or adversity and include the following:

- Reactive Attachment Disorder
- Disinhibited Social Engagement Disorder
- PTSD
- Acute Stress Disorder
- Adjustment Disorder
- Other Specified Trauma- and Stressor-Related Disorder
- Unspecified Trauma- and Stressor-Related Disorder

As described in Chapter 1, children exposed to developmental adversity, especially repeated exposure or exposure to varied adversities, can experience many symptoms, resulting in the clinician giving the child several diagnoses. According to Berliner et al. (2020), differential diagnosis and the presence of co-occurring disorders need to be entertained because behavioral health disorders have a higher base rate in trauma-exposed children and adolescents, and comorbidity of conditions occurs more often than not (Lewis et al., 2019). When the treatment setting requires a documented diagnosis (e.g., for payment of services by a health insurance company), diagnosing the child with multiple diagnoses initially provides clerical utility but not necessarily clinical usefulness. Such a situation is particularly challenging when the number of diagnoses becomes unwieldy—usually more than four disorders. In this case, focusing on spheres or domains of dysfunction is arguably more clinically relevant than emphasizing numerous diagnoses containing many symptoms. Targeting areas of dysfunction would be clinically indicated and acceptable in settings where diagnoses are not required. As a reminder, the domains of dysfunction in the proposed diagnosis, DTD, are apropos to this discussion (i.e., emotion dysregulation, behavior and attention dysregulation, and self and relational dysregulation). However, until DTD becomes recognized as an "official" diagnosis (e.g., appearing in the next iteration of the *Diagnostic and Statistical Manual of Mental Disorders* [DSM]), determining acceptable diagnoses for treatment planning purposes is the conventional way to proceed.

The clinician can use the Treatment Planning Form to develop a comprehensive and personalized treatment plan for the child (see Appendix B). As outlined, the form comprises the major sections described above—long-term goals, short-term objectives, interventions, and diagnosis. In addition, templates to define goals and objectives are also included to guide the clinician in writing the targets for treatment in an individualized manner. The following plan was created for a hypothetical child who will provide the basis for the remainder of this manual to fully illustrate how the clinician can utilize the Treatment Planning Form. A description of the child and the reason for referral and initial clinical presentation will then be provided. This information will be followed by an illustration of the conducted assessments and corresponding findings. The case conceptualization will then be presented, including the clinical formulation (i.e., primary problems, 3 Ps, and theory) and treatment-related factors (i.e., personal strengths, external resources, and problems). This entire clinical picture of the child consequently sets the stage for Chapter 5—parent training to help their child enhance their emotion regulation skills.

Treatment Plan for Lucas (An Example)

Long-Term Goals

1) At the end of treatment, when Lucas is triggered by his mother when he is told to do his homework, especially math, he reacts by engaging less in behavioral avoidance of the work; loud, angry verbal refusal (e.g., *"I hate math!"*); and running away (i.e., out of the family's apartment to the stairwell down the hall). As a result, Lucas experiences greater participation in doing his homework, particularly math-related learning tasks. This increased engagement puts him at higher chances for academic progress and success.

2) At the end of treatment, when Lucas is triggered by his brother or sister (or peer at school) when he is either not asked to join them in an activity or is told that he is not allowed to participate, he reacts by engaging less in social withdrawal and isolation. As a result, Lucas experiences greater participation in other social interactions and activities. This increased engagement puts him at higher chances of improving his social development.

3) At the end of treatment, when Lucas is triggered by loud voices of others (or loud sounds in general), he reacts by engaging less in escape behavior and

shutting down (i.e., crawling into his bed, pulling the covers over his head, and quietly crying). As a result, Lucas experiences greater participation in independent and family-based activities. This increased engagement puts him at higher chances for positive interactions and relationships with his mother, brother, and sister.

Short-Term Objectives

1) After one month of treatment, when Lucas is triggered by his mother when he is told to do his homework, especially math, he reacts by engaging 25% less in behavioral avoidance of the work, loud, angry verbal refusal, and running away. As a result, Lucas experiences 25% greater participation in frequency in doing his homework.
2) After one month of treatment, when Lucas is triggered by his brother or sister (or peer at school) when he is either not asked to join them in an activity or is told that he's not allowed to participate, he reacts by engaging 25% less in social withdrawal and isolation. As a result, Lucas experiences 25% greater participation in frequency in other social interactions and activities.
3) After one month of treatment, when Lucas is triggered by loud voices of others (or loud sounds in general), he reacts by engaging 25% less in escape behavior and shutting down (i.e., crawling into his bed, pulling the covers over his head, and crying quietly). As a result, Lucas experiences 25% greater participation in frequency in independent and family-based activities.

Interventions (at Least One for Each Objective)

1) Trauma-Informed Parenting Program (TIP^s); cognitive restructuring; referral for psychopharmacology
2) TIP^s
3) TIP^s; exposure work; referral for psychopharmacology

Diagnosis

1) Post-Traumatic Stress Disorder (if a formal DSM/ICD diagnosis is required)
2) DTD

Reason for Referral

Lucas's mother, Adriana, was referred to a behavioral healthcare clinician within the pediatric integrated care department of a local community health center when she brought him in for what was eventually diagnosed as an ear infection. At that time, she reported that he was having emotional and behavioral problems at home and in school. Lucas told the primary care provider, *"I get really mad sometimes."*

Background Information

Lucas is a nine-year-old, cis-gender, Brazilian-American male in the 3rd grade at a local elementary school. He currently lives with his biological mother, Adriana, and his 12-year-old brother and younger sister, who is eight years old. His father, Francisco, lives on the other side of town with a 1st-degree cousin. He moved out of the family's apartment about six months ago when Adriana told him to leave once she could no longer take his reported escalating alcohol use problem and verbal abuse toward her and the children.

Lucas's parents moved to the United States from Brazil when his brother was two years old. They had both been working in the food industry for many years—he as a head cook at a local restaurant, and she also as a cook in the cafeteria of a local hospital. Although Adriana was able to keep her job after the onset of the COVID-19 pandemic, Francisco ended up losing his job because the restaurant owner where he worked went out of business due to the pandemic. Because virtually no restaurants were hiring new staff, he could not find a job as a cook. Therefore, he became a food delivery driver for DoorDash.

Both of Lucas's parents have histories of behavioral health problems. Adriana reported a chronic history of a generalized anxiety problem. Before the pandemic, Francisco already had an alcohol use problem, to which Lucas was exposed for several years, and a history of a depression problem. He also would become verbally abusive toward Adriana when he was under the influence of excess alcohol. Lucas, unfortunately, witnessed this behavior on many occasions. When Francisco became a driver, his workdays typically started in the late afternoon. Combined with the requirement to remain inside due to the widespread lockdowns resulting from the pandemic, the extended amount of time Francisco stayed in the apartment led him to drink more alcohol. Lucas was also at home most of the time as school became completely remote, but his mother continued to go to the hospital for work. Lucas and his siblings were repeatedly verbally abused by Francisco before leaving the apartment for his driving job. At the time of the referral, Lucas had rare and inconsistent contact with his father. Reportedly, Francisco "just shows up" at the family's apartment demanding to see Lucas and his siblings and "acts drunk."

Assessment Findings

The clinician interviewed Adriana using the Trauma Event Screening Instrument for Children (Ribbe, 1996), Child PTSD Symptom Scale for DSM-5 (Foa et al., 2018), DTD Semi-Structured Interview (Ford et al., 2018), and the Child and Adolescent Functional Assessment Scale (Hodges, 2000a; 2000b). They also asked her to complete several rating scales, including the UCLA PTSD Reaction Index (Kaplow et al., 2020), Coronavirus Impact Scale

(Stoddard et al. 2021), and the Emotion Regulation Checklist (Shields and Cicchetti, 1997). In addition, Lucas filled out Perceptions of Racism in Children and Youth (Pachter et al., 2010) and the Child Post-Traumatic Cognitions Inventory (Meiser-Stedman et al., 2009).

The assessment results indicate that Lucas has been exposed to multiple developmental adversities. Specifically, he has been raised in a family in which both parents have behavioral health problems (otherwise known as "impaired caregivers" using ACE Study terminology). He also has endured years of verbal abuse from his father. In addition, his father being "kicked out" of the home by his mother and the resulting lack of contact with his father are further adversities. Furthermore, Lucas endorsed being a survivor of racial/ethnic discrimination, such as being called an insulting name, hearing someone making a negative or insulting remark about his ethnicity, and seeing his parents treated unfairly or badly because of their accent or origin from a different country. Lastly, he (and his family) has been exposed to pandemic-related adverse experiences, including reduced family income, decreased access to social supports, elevated stress and discord in the family, and having an extended family member diagnosed with COVID-19.

The assessment findings also indicate various symptoms, problems, dysregulation, and impairment. Notably, Lucas presently has several post-traumatic stress symptoms: emotional distress after exposure to traumatic reminders, negative affect, irritability, risky behavior, and difficulty concentrating. He also presents with adversity-related maladaptive cognitions. Regarding regulatory processes, he evidently has problems across the three domains of the DTD diagnosis, namely affective and physiological, behavioral and attentional, and self and relational dysregulation. According to the Child and Adolescent Functional Assessment Scale results, Lucas is impaired in the following life areas: school, home, community, behavior toward others, and moods/emotions.

Three patterns emerged from the assessment of emotion dysregulation episodes. First, being told to do his homework by his mother elicits a dysregulated state that includes potentially dangerous behavior—running out of the family's apartment to the stairwell down the hall. This dysregulation is evidently associated with the school-related verbal abuse that Lucas endured from his father during remote learning in the early part of the pandemic, such as being called *stupid, lazy,* and *idiot.* A second pattern appears connected to Lucas feeling rejected, which occurs when a sibling or school peer doesn't ask him to join an activity or is told that he is not allowed to participate. Again, this dysregulation is likely related to his father in that he would often ignore and not include Lucas when under the influence of alcohol. Lastly, a pattern of dysregulation is present that is triggered by loud voices or sounds in general. This dysregulated state is apparently associated with his father's naturally booming and projecting voice, which would become amplified whenever he drank alcohol and became angry.

Case Conceptualization

Clinical Formulation
Lucas is exhibiting three primary problems. First, when Lucas is triggered by his mother when he is told to do his homework, especially math, he reacts by engaging in behavioral avoidance of the work; loud, angry verbal refusal (e.g., *"I hate math!"*); and running away (i.e., out of the family's apartment to the stairwell down the hall). As a result, Lucas experiences less participation in doing his homework, particularly math-related learning tasks. This decreased engagement puts him at risk for academic problems. Second, when Lucas is triggered by his brother or sister (or peer at school) when he is either not asked to join them in an activity or is told that he is not allowed to participate, he reacts by engaging in social withdrawal and isolation. As a result, Lucas experiences less participation in other social interactions and activities. This decreased engagement puts him at risk for problems in his social development. Third, when Lucas is triggered by loud voices of others (or loud sounds in general), he reacts by engaging in escape behavior and shutting down (i.e., crawling into his bed, pulling the covers over his head, and quietly crying). As a result, Lucas experiences less participation in independent and family-based activities. This decreased engagement puts him at risk for negative interactions and relationships with his mother, brother, and sister.

Several factors have contributed to the onset and maintenance of Lucas's problems. Predispositions include a significant family history of behavioral health problems and, relatedly, his parents being impaired caregivers. Exposure to his father verbally abusing his mother was also a predisposing factor. Presumed atypical neurodevelopment associated with his exposure to ACEs is another predisposition. Precipitants to his problems were multiple: stressors related to the COVID-19 pandemic; household financial stress due to his father losing his job; verbal abuse by his father; his parents' ongoing impaired caregiver status; as well as his father leaving the family home and the resulting minimal contact with him. Lucas's poor emotion regulation skills and maladaptive cognitions most likely perpetuate his problems. Through the lens of cognitive theory, he is predicted to have a sense of ongoing threat within his environment. This perception, in turn, is prolonged by negative appraisals of his exposure to developmental adversity and post-adversity experiences, as well as poorly integrated or elaborated memories of the ACEs he has endured. Lucas likely also has maladaptive cognitive coping strategies.

Treatment-Related Factors
Lucas possesses several personal strengths. He is friendly and likable. Although he tends to withdraw, Lucas is sociable and prefers the presence of others. He seems to be above average in regard to psychological mindedness and insight. Despite his chronic environmental challenges at home, he has been

able to succeed academically (at least until recently), and his intellectual abilities are estimated to be average to above average. Last year, Lucas began playing soccer, which he enjoys and has talent. His reported desire and commitment to learning how to play better by improving his skillset may translate to putting in the time and effort needed to enhance his emotion regulation capacity. External resources include his mother, who strives to do and wants the best for Lucas and his siblings; his mother's best friend and family (they live in the same apartment building as Lucas); his teacher; and his soccer coach. Problems that may hinder Lucas's participation in and benefit from treatment are the absence of his father, limited transportation (his father has the family's only car), and restricted childcare options for Lucas's siblings when Lucas (with his mother) or his mother alone needs to leave their home for treatment.

Trauma-Informed Parenting Program (*TIP[s] for Clinicians*): An Introduction

In Chapter 5, a complete protocol is outlined for the clinician to work with the parent to improve their child's emotion regulation skills. Lucas and his mother will be used to illustrate how this work is conducted. The first part of the training will focus on the clinician working with both of them to teach Lucas emotion identification skills in tandem with his mother. This aspect is grounded in our understanding of emotions, as highlighted in Chapter 3. As a reminder, regularity typically exists between the perceived stimulus and the resulting emotion elicited and experienced, such as a source of perceived threat triggering the emotion that we identify as anxiety. Besides covering the basic emotions (and perhaps more complex ones depending on the child's age), a sufficient number of exemplars will be reviewed so that Lucas and his mother will know with confidence the patterns between specific emotional stimuli and their corresponding emotions. Second, the clinician will work solely with Lucas's mother to train her how to teach Lucas emotion regulation skills. As described previously, these skills comprise tracking, evaluating, and altering emotions so that the child can accomplish their goals or meet the demands of the present environment (Thompson, 1994). Given that parents can be their children's best and most influential teachers, training parents to teach their children how to improve their emotion regulation and related behavior can have a substantial and long-standing impact on their overall development. This work is what lies next.

5

Guidelines for Clinicians

At the end of this chapter, you will be able to:

- Explain to children exposed to developmental adversity that emotion dys-regulation underlies their misbehavior, acting out, and withdrawal
- Teach children the main components of emotions
- Help children learn the regularity of and specificity between emotional stimuli and elicited emotions
- Train parents how to teach their children emotion regulation skills
  - o Emotion modulation skills
  - o Cognitive reappraisal/restructuring skills
  - o Problem-solving skills

TIP^s for the Treatment Plan

This chapter is all about putting the treatment plan into action. As we learned in Chapter 4, the Trauma-Informed Parenting Program (*TIP^s for Clinicians*) is essentially an integration of two of the four common intervention elements found in science-based treatments—coping skills and parenting support and skills (Jensen et al., 2020). *TIP^s* also incorporates the features and tenets of successful parent training models (Shaffer et al., 2001). Precisely, *TIP^s* has a primary focus on parents instead of children. This emphasis aligns with acknowledging the importance of intervening at the level of the system—in this case, the family system. The treatment stresses enhancing an integral regulatory process rather than decreasing symptoms and problems. Although symptom reduction is an important outcome, improved adaptive functioning takes precedence. Teaching parents to target behavioral indicators is paramount because behavior is concrete, objective, operationally definable, and therefore measurable. Training new parenting skills (e.g., use of reinforcement, generalization of skills across settings) and addressing factors that may negatively impact treatment and outcomes are also critical components of *TIP^s*. Collectively, the treatment brings these characteristics together to maximize its effects. The overarching goal is to improve the child's behavioral health, hopefully leading to a richer and more meaningful life.

Part I: Teaching Emotion Identification Skills

The first part of TIP^s is focused on teaching the child and parent emotion identification skills. Thus, treatment sessions include the child-parent dyad. If the family unit comprises two parents, then their simultaneous participation is highly encouraged. However, real-world practice and experience dictate that the presence of only one parent in treatment is the rule rather than the exception. Although this situation also exists with single-parent households, one parent's engagement in treatment typically occurs even when joint legal (but sole physical) custody is in place. Regardless, initial work with the dyad during the first couple sessions centers on our understanding of the primary goal that effective emotion regulation is dependent on what the child can do for themselves when experiencing an emotion (i.e., intrinsic processes) as well as what the parent can do if they are present at the moment (i.e., extrinsic processes). The following script highlights how the first session unfolds.

Session 1 - Introduction to Emotion Identification Training

At the end of the session, the child and parent will be able to:

- Understand that very stressful experiences during childhood (i.e., exposure to developmental adversity) have negative effects on a person's health and development
- Know that how the brain develops is impacted by ACEs, which affects how children cope with their emotions, especially their negative ones
- Know the fundamental characteristics of emotions
- Begin the between-session work of emotion identification training

CLINICIAN: *Hi Lucas and Adriana. It's great to see you. I hope that everything's been OK since our last meeting* (intake assessment). *Today, I want to talk about and work on what we call emotions or feelings with both of you. This work is very important because of what you've gone through, Lucas, the past few years, and how you're handling your emotions now. What I mean is that when I met with you and your mom, I learned that many bad or negative things have happened in your life, especially with your dad, that have affected how you've grown and developed. Those things or experiences I'm talking about are your dad's drinking and problems with alcohol; his meanness and anger towards you, your mom, and your sister and brother; him moving out of your home and living somewhere else; and you not being able to see your dad and hang out with him. Also, we've all been going through the COVID-19 pandemic, and my understanding is that it's affected you and your family in negative ways. Do either of you have any questions so far?*

ADRIANA: *What do you mean that the things you just said have had a negative effect on Lucas?*

CLINICIAN: *Great question, Adriana! A simple way to think about it is that those situations or experiences have been very stressful for Lucas, and really for your entire family, and that they were the causes or sources of the stress that he has gone through. We also know from scientific research that although some stress is OK, a lot of stress is bad for our health and development. And it doesn't matter if you're a kid, teenager, or adult. What about you, Lucas? Do you have any questions?*

LUCAS: *So, is there something wrong with me because of this stuff that you just said?*

CLINICIAN: *Absolutely not, Lucas! What I want you to know is that this stuff has made it harder or more challenging for you to handle difficult situations. The things that have happened with your dad have probably affected how your brain has developed* (Clinician points to their head). *Because your brain controls your emotions and pretty much everything about you, that's why you get really mad sometimes and don't know what to do in those situations. Make sense, Lucas?*

LUCAS: *Uh-huh* (Lucas nods his head "yes").

CLINICIAN: *Besides getting mad or angry, I also learned from you and your mom that you have other emotions that you have a hard time dealing with. Isn't that right, Adriana?*

ADRIANA: *Yes, you're right. Not only does Lucas get really mad, he can feel very nervous and sad too.*

CLINICIAN: *Can you give me an example, Adriana?*

ADRIANA: *Well, when Lucas wants to play with his brother or sister, but they don't want to, he gets quite sad and disappears to his bedroom for a long time.*

CLINICIAN: *Did what your mom say sound right, Lucas?*

LUCAS: *I guess so. I don't like it when my sister or brother doesn't want to play with me.*

CLINICIAN: *Then, you go to your bedroom?*

LUCAS: *Uh-huh.*

CLINICIAN: *What do you do in there?*

LUCAS: *Nothing really. I just hang out until my mom tells me to come out.*

CLINICIAN: *What do you have to add to what Lucas just said, Adriana?*

ADRIANA: *Lucas is mostly right. Whenever I notice that Lucas isn't in the kitchen or family room, I go and check the bedroom he shares with his brother. He usually says that he's OK and that he's just playing by himself. But, I can see that he's really not doing anything in there and that he's feeling sad, which makes me figure out that his brother and sister don't want to play with him. I then leave him alone until it's time for him to come out, such as for lunch or dinner or when I need to take him and his sister with me for an errand.*

CLINICIAN: *Adriana, do you know if something like this happens to Lucas at school?*

ADRIANA: *Lucas's teacher emailed me a few weeks ago to tell me that he's become more and more worried about him. He said that Lucas has been spending a lot of time alone during recess and not playing with his classmates.*

CLINICIAN: *I understand. Thank you both for explaining to me what happens when you, Lucas, have a hard time dealing with things at home and in school. Now, let me tell you what I think is going on in these situations. First, something happens that you see as negative or bad, Lucas, which then makes you feel a certain emotion, such as feeling sad—the emotion that we call "sadness." You sometimes might also feel a couple of emotions at the same time. Second, the emotion that you feel is usually too strong for you to handle, and you don't know what to do about it or the situation. Third, because you're not sure what to do, you end up doing something else instead and not what you want to be doing or are supposed to be doing.*

So, the main goal of our work together is for you, Lucas, to be able to handle or deal with your emotions better in the future so that you end up doing what you want or need to do, such as playing with your classmates and working on school assignments. Sometimes, I'll use the words, "cope" and "regulate," when I'm talking about how people can change parts of their emotions, such as how strong they are or when they happen. One impor- tant way that I want you to think about this work is that you'll <u>learn how to make yourself feel better when you're feeling emotionally bad or negative on the inside.</u> However, before you can cope with or regulate your emotions, you have to be able to identify what specific emotion or emotions you're feeling or experiencing. This ability is called emotion identification skills. So, we'll all work together for a couple of *meetings so that you and your mom get really good at identifying many of your emotions and what kinds of situations are connected to them. Then, I'll work just with you, Adriana, to teach you how to teach Lucas to better regulate his emotions at home. We'll also figure out ways to help you, Lucas, better deal or cope with your emotions in school too. But, before we move on, I want to know if this sounds good to you, Lucas, and if you do really want to learn how to handle or regulate your emotions better.*

LUCAS: *I do.*

CLINICIAN: *How about you, Adriana? Does everything make sense, and do you want to do this work to help Lucas?*

ADRIANA: *Definitely! I want Lucas to be happy, to have friends to play with, and to do well in school.*

At this point in the session, the clinician has conveyed the following information:

- Exposure to developmental adversity negatively affects the child's health and development.
- Adverse childhood experiences (ACEs) specifically impact the brain and the child's ability to regulate emotions
- Emotion dysregulation interferes with the child's goals or meeting the demands of the environment

Before continuing, the clinician then established an initial treatment alliance by getting an agreement among the three of them on the overarching target for change (i.e., emotion dysregulation) and the corresponding intervention (i.e., *TIP^s*). At the outset of therapeutic work, the treatment alliance provides a cornerstone of engaging and retaining children and families impacted by developmental adversity in treatment (Saxe et al., 2012). From here, the clinician introduces training in emotion identification skills.

CLINICIAN: *To start, do you know what emotions are, Lucas?*

LUCAS: *Our feelings, right?*

CLINICIAN: *That's correct, Lucas. All people have or experience what we call feelings or emotions, and it doesn't matter if you're a kid, teenager, or adult, like your mom and me. Everyone has emotions because they are part of being human. Now, I'm wondering if you can think of and name an emotion, Lucas.*

LUCAS: *Happy?*

CLINICIAN: *Right again! When we feel happy, we experience the emotion called "happiness." This emotion is the number one or most important positive emotion. The word, "positive," is used to mean that the emotion feels good on the inside. People usually have positive emotions when things are going their way or turning out the way they want them to. Can you think of a time recently when you felt happy or experienced the emotion, "happiness," Lucas?*

LUCAS: *Well, I was happy when my mom took me to my favorite playground last weekend, and I got to play with my best friend.*

CLINICIAN: *What a great example, Lucas! It sounds like you had lots of fun. I really like this example because I can completely understand what made you feel happy in that situation. The main thing I want you to know and remember is that happiness is the positive emotion people feel when they get what they want. In this case, my guess is that you wanted to go to your favorite playground and that you wanted to play with your best friend.*

LUCAS: *Uh-huh.*

CLINICIAN: *I thought so. Now, let's bring your mom into the conversation. Adriana, I'm wondering how you would feel emotionally if you went to one of your favorite places, like a restaurant, and were able to eat and hang out there with one of your best friends.*

ADRIANA: *I would feel happy too.*

CLINICIAN: *I bet! My best understanding is that pretty much everyone in the world would feel happy or experience happiness if they got to go to one of their favorite places and hang out or do stuff with their best friend. What I want both of you to learn from these examples is that emotions have patterns to them—certain situations lead to certain emotions. In this situation, Lucas, you wanted something and got it—playing with your best friend at your favorite playground. And remember, happiness is the emotion people feel when they get what they want. Let's look at another example. Is there something that you wanted recently and got, Adriana?*

ADRIANA: *I wanted Lucas to do well on his last math homework assignment, and he got a B+.*

CLINICIAN: *Good for you, Lucas! Did you want to do well on that assignment?*

LUCAS: *I sure did.*

CLINICIAN: *Because you got want you wanted, how did it make you feel?*

LUCAS: *Happy.*

CLINICIAN: *Awesome! To repeat, we feel happy when we get what we want. As it turns out, the other main positive emotions are pretty similar to happiness. These emotions include joy and satisfaction. So, all positive emotions are something people feel when things are going well or going their way. In other words, we feel good on the inside when things are going right or turning out the way we want them to.*

To review, here is what was covered in this part of the session:

- Emotions are fundamental to being human, and that one major category of emotions is experienced as feeling positive
- Happiness is the prototypical positive emotion
- The child was able to identify an activity, event, or situation that recently elicited happiness, which the clinician verbally reinforced
- Feeling happy typically results when people get what they want
- The parent was brought into the conversation by being asked to share a recent experience that elicited happiness in them, which also triggered the child to feel happy too because both wanted the same thing—doing well on a school assignment
- Emotions were described to have patterns in that specific ones are usually elicited by certain types of situations (i.e., sources of emotional stimulation)
- Other fundamental positive emotions are merely extensions of happiness and thus result when wants or needs are obtained

The next section of the session introduces negative emotions. In this phase, the child learns specifics about their challenging emotional experiences.

CLINICIAN: *Now, we're going to switch to talking about negative emotions. These emotional experiences are labeled as negative because they make people feel "bad" or not good on the inside. People usually feel emotionally bad or negative when things are going wrong. As an example, I'm wondering if you, Lucas, know what the emotion, "sadness," is and if you can think of a time when you recently felt sad.*

LUCAS: *I was sad when my dad moved out of our apartment.*

CLINICIAN: *And how did you feel on the inside?*

LUCAS: *Bad. Really bad.*

CLINICIAN: *Now, I feel badly for you knowing that you had to go through that experience.*

LUCAS: *Yeah. It sucks that my dad doesn't live with us anymore.*

CLINICIAN: *I hear you, Lucas. But, I also want to tell you that the situation with your dad that you just came up with is a great example for our conversation about negative emotions. In this case, you felt sad or experienced the emotion, sadness, because you "lost" someone, but not forever like when somebody you know dies. What I mean is that you've lost chances to see and do things with your dad because he's not living with you. Overall, sadness is what we usually feel when we lose someone or something that's part of our lives. And the more important that person or thing is to us, the sadder we feel when we lose them. Another reason that this example is a really good one is because most people would feel sad if someone important to them moved away. I'm wondering if you've ever experienced this situation, Adriana.*

ADRIANA: *Of course! When I was in grade school in Brazil, one of my best friends moved away to another city, which was a very sad situation for me.*

CLINICIAN: *You mean that you felt quite sad when that happened?*

ADRIANA: *Yes. I did.*

CLINICIAN: *Thanks for sharing that experience, Adriana. So, just like the emotion, happiness, sadness also has a typical pattern—we usually feel sad when we lose something or someone important to us. Put another way, a loss can make or trigger people to feel sad. Have you recently lost something important to you, Adriana?*

ADRIANA: *Unfortunately, I lost an earring of one of my favorite pairs, and I definitely felt sad afterwards for a while.*

CLINICIAN: *How about you, Lucas?*

LUCAS: *I don't think I've lost anything lately.*

CLINICIAN: *Can you think of something that's yours that would make you feel sad if you lost it?*

LUCAS: *Uhm, a Razor scooter that used to be my brother's.*

CLINICIAN: *Razors are cool! I can imagine you feeling really sad if you lost your scooter. Hopefully, you won't ever lose it.*
Let's now talk about another negative emotion before we end today's meeting. That emotion is called "anger"—in other words, feeling angry or mad. My guess is that you have a pretty good idea what this emotion is all about, Lucas.

LUCAS: *Uh-huh. Sometimes, I get really mad.*

CLINICIAN: *Can you give an example?*

LUCAS: *When my mother makes me do my homework.*

CLINICIAN: *That example is really a perfect one, Lucas, because anger is an emotion we usually feel towards someone when that person doesn't give us what we want or gets in our way, like our parents or brothers and sisters too* (and generically "siblings" if gender neutrality is present as part of someone's identity). *In other words, anger is the opposite of happiness because, as we talked about a few minutes ago, we feel happy when we do get what we want or that things are turning out the way we want them to. Does that make sense?*

ADRIANA: *I thought feeling sad was the opposite of happy.*

CLINICIAN: *Well, many, if not most, people think that way. But, I want you and Lucas to focus on is thinking about the emotions backwards in time. The first step is to identify what specific emotion or emotions you're currently feeling. Once you figure out what that is, then the second step is to think about what certain activity, event, or situation happened before you started feeling the emotion. In other words, emotions are felt after situations occur and usually immediately afterward or right away. To repeat, anger (or feeling angry or mad) happens after we don't get what we want; sadness or feeling sad is what we experience after we lose something or someone, and happiness is the feeling we have after we get what we want.*

ADRIANA: *OK. That makes sense, then.*

CLINICIAN: *Do you have any questions, Lucas?*

LUCAS: *Nuh-uh* (Lucas shakes his head "no").

CLINICIAN: *So, before we end today's meeting, I want to tell you about an activity I want you to do, Lucas, before our next meeting. Like you told me before, you do want to learn how to handle or regulate your emotions better. For this to happen, you need to first practice identifying your emotions and the situations connected to them; and the more you practice, the better you'll get. This week, I want you to work on the emotions of anger and sadness. Let me show you this worksheet I want you to fill out for this activity* (Clinician pulls out the Emotion Identification Worksheet (see Appendix C)). *Here, you can see that the worksheet is divided into rows and that each row has three parts. I want you to fill out a row when you've experienced or felt an emotion. For each row, start by writing down in the middle part the emotion you identified that you felt, either anger or sadness. Then, write down on the left side of the row the situation that happened right before you felt the emotion. Do you have any questions so far, Lucas?*

LUCAS: *I don't think so.*

CLINICIAN: *Great! The last part is to write on the right side of the row what you did while you were feeling angry or sad. This is how you behaved with your actions and words.*

LUCAS: *Do I have to do this worksheet by myself?*

CLINICIAN: *If you think that you can finish a whole row by yourself, then do it. But I expect there'll be times when you're going to want to ask your mom for help, which is just fine. My guess is that you'll need help the most for the last part of each row where you have to write down how you acted when feeling angry or sad. Adriana, when Lucas asks you to help him figure out what he did, I want you to ask him two questions: 1) "What did you do that someone could see?" and 2) "What did you say that someone could hear?" In other words, if you can see it or hear it, that's behavior or a person's actions.*

Also, when you notice, Adriana, that Lucas is feeling angry or sad during the week, I want you to ask him afterward if he filled out one of the rows. If he says "yes" and shows you the worksheet, then I want you to offer him a reward, or reinforcement, for completing the row. The reward should be small and easy to give, such as an extra afternoon snack, a bigger dessert after dinner, or a couple extra minutes of "fun time" at night before getting ready for bed. Of course, I also want you to reward Lucas for completing a row and showing you the worksheet when he does so without you asking him. Are you willing to do this, Adriana?

ADRIANA: *For sure!*

CLINICIAN: *That's great because not only do I want you to show him with rewards that this activity is important to you, but also that these rewards will hopefully motivate him to complete the worksheet. Is that right, Lucas?*

LUCAS: *Uh-huh.*

CLINICIAN: *Perfect! One last thing—just try your best and don't worry about doing it right or wrong, Lucas. If you practice enough times, you'll end up getting it and being able to use this skill in identifying emotions for your whole life. As I often say, "Practice makes permanent."*

To review, here is what was covered in this last part of the session:

- Negative emotions were introduced as experiences that feel "bad" internally and generally result from the failure of attaining wants and needs
- The child was able to identify an activity, event, or situation that recently elicited a specific negative emotion, sadness, which the clinician verbally reinforced
- Feeling sad typically results when people lose something or someone important to them
- The parent was brought into the conversation by being asked to share experiences that elicited sadness in them
- The child was able to identify an activity, event, or situation that recently elicited a different negative emotion, anger, which the clinician verbally reinforced
- Feeling angry typically results when someone interferes with getting our wants and needs met
- Emotions can be accurately identified by working "backwards" to find the activity, event, or situation that elicited them beforehand in time
- Between-session work was described, and the Emotion Identification Worksheet was introduced and reviewed
- Behavior was simply defined by its visual and auditory characteristics
- The use of reinforcement by the parent was introduced as a means to facilitate and motivate the child's learning

Session 2 - Continuation of Emotion Identification Training and Introduction to Emotion Regulation Training

At the end of the session, the child and parent will be able to:

- Understand that negative emotions typically motivate people to act in ways to decrease or eliminate the associated, internal "bad" feeling
- Know that such emotion-motivated behavior can interfere with achieving goals or meeting the demands of the environment
- Understand that the "bad" feeling of negative emotions can be reduced by engaging in acceptable and appropriate behavior that elicits internal positivity
- Begin the between-session work of emotion regulation training when the child is well-regulated

CLINICIAN: *Hi Lucas and Adriana. It's nice to see you again. I hope that you and your family have been doing well since our last meeting. I'm excited to hear if you, Lucas, were able to work on that activity and complete the Emotion Identification Worksheet.*

ADRIANA: *Lucas did a great job! Although he earned rewards just like you told me to give him, he really didn't need them because he wants to learn to be well-behaved.*

CLINICIAN: *Is that right, Lucas?*

LUCAS: *I don't want to get as mad as I do and make my mom upset.*

CLINICIAN: *That sounds like an important goal to you, Lucas, and probably something that your mom wants too.*

ADRIANA: Adriana nods her head in agreement.

CLINICIAN: *So, let's see what you filled out on the worksheet* (Adriana pulls out the paper from her purse). *It looks like you completed a few of these rows. I agree with your mom—what a great job you did! Now, I want to hear and learn about a couple of these situations from you. I'll let you pick. What situation do you want to talk about first?*

LUCAS: *My mom said that I should talk about how I hate doing homework.*

CLINICIAN: *OK. Well, it looks like this row here is about your homework, and you wrote down the word, angry, in the middle part* (the Clinician points to that section of the worksheet). *What was the situation that made you feel the emotion, anger, Lucas?*

LUCAS: *My mom asked me if I finished my homework and to show her what I did. When I pulled it out of my backpack, she looked at it and asked if I had any math to do. I said, "Yes." Then, she asked if I did it because she didn't see anything with math on it. When I said, "No," she told me that I had to do it right away.*

CLINICIAN: *I think I get it. So, what happened next? Here, you wrote the word "stairs"* (the Clinician points to that section of the worksheet).

LUCAS: *I left our apartment and went to the stairs at the end of the hall.*

ADRIANA: *He also said, "I hate math," and actually ran down the hall to the stairs.*

CLINICIAN: *What happened after that?*

LUCAS: *My mom came and got me.*

ADRIANA: *I followed Lucas right away and sat next to him at the top of the stairs, which is where he usually goes. I reminded him that he just needs to try his best with his homework and that I'll help him any time he wants me to or when he needs it. His dad used to get extremely angry at him when he couldn't do his homework by himself and would ask for help, especially with math because that's his hardest subject.*

CLINICIAN: *I understand. Let me say a couple things before we move on. First, I'm proud of you, Lucas, for doing this activity and completing the worksheet. As I told you before, the more you practice and do the work, the better you'll get at knowing what your emotions are and then learning how to change or regulate them. Second, you should be proud of yourself, Lucas, for doing such a great job with this activity and worksheet. Third, this example of you getting angry is a really good one for me to better understand what can make you feel this emotion. But, I do have a couple of questions. When you got angry after your mom told you to do your math homework, I'm wondering how angry did you get? A little angry, really angry, or somewhere in the middle?*

LUCAS: *Really angry.*

CLINICIAN: *Thanks for letting me know. Do you remember, Lucas, when do people usually feel the emotion, anger?*

LUCAS: *Nuh-uh.*

CLINICIAN: *People usually feel angry when they don't get what they want. Do you remember that, Lucas?*

LUCAS: *Yes.*

CLINICIAN: *So, when people feel really angry, that usually means that they didn't get what they really wanted. What did you really want in that situation, Lucas?*

LUCAS: *I really didn't want to do my math homework.*

CLINICIAN: *Another way to say that is that you really wanted to not do or skip your math homework. Does that make sense?*

LUCAS: *Uh-huh. I don't want to do any math homework at all!*

CLINICIAN: *It sounds like math is definitely not your favorite subject! So, when you felt really angry after your mom told you to do your math homework right away, you ran down the hall to the stairs instead.*

Well, that behavior makes sense to me because the emotion, anger, and other negative emotions usually drive or motivate us to do something to decrease how strong the emotion is or to make the emotion go away altogether. Another thing that we sometimes do is to try and make whatever made us feel this way stop or go away, such as someone who did or said something to us. One other thing that we can do is just leave ourselves. In this situation, Lucas, you went away from your mom after she told you to do your math homework.

LUCAS: *But, I ended up finishing my homework.*

CLINICIAN: *And that's great, Lucas! However, before you finished your homework, you left the apartment by yourself, which is an unsafe or dangerous thing to do. Isn't that right, Adriana?*

ADRIANA: *You know that I never want you to leave the apartment alone. Don't you, Lucas?*

LUCAS: Lucas nods his head "yes."

CLINICIAN: *Then, do you want to learn how to control or regulate your anger so that you don't leave the apartment by yourself anymore?*

LUCAS: Lucas again nods his head "yes."

CLINICIAN: *That's great, Lucas! That will be the next part of our work together.*

To review, here is what was covered in this first part of the session:

- The clinician confirmed that the child completed the emotion identification activity and associated worksheet
- With the aid of the worksheet, the child was able to identify a situation that elicited a negative emotion, anger, to a significant degree
- The parent was encouraged to add clarifying information, which included the child engaging in dangerous behavior and how this situation is related to exposure to emotional abuse by his father
- The clinician reminded the child and parent that anger is an emotional reaction to not getting what we want or need
- The clinician described that anger and other negative emotions typically motivate people to act in ways to decrease the internal experience or to be removed from the person who was the source of emotional stimulation
- The clinician described how this experience was an episode of emotion dysregulation due to the intensity of the anger and the resulting behavior
- The clinician confirmed that the parent wants the behavior to change (i.e., eliminated) and that the child wants to learn how to effect this modification

The next section of the session reviews another episode, but with a different emotion (sadness) and emotion-related behavior.

CLINICIAN: *Let's talk about another situation that you filled out on the worksheet. I see here that you wrote down the word, "sad." Can you see what you wrote down on the left side of the row* (Clinician points to that section of the worksheet)*?*

LUCAS: *"Leo" and "video game."*

CLINICIAN: *Did you write those words down all by yourself?*

LUCAS: *I asked my mom to help me spell them.*

CLINICIAN: *Perfect, Lucas! So, what do you remember about that situation?*

LUCAS: *Leo didn't let me play video games with him.*

CLINICIAN: *Because your brother didn't want to play with you, you ended up feeling the emotion, sadness, and you wrote the word ,"sad," in the middle part of the row. Then, it looks like you wrote: "went to bedroom." What did you do in your bedroom?*

LUCAS: *I don't know.*

ADRIANA: *I remember going to his room to check on him, and he was just sitting next to the window looking outside.*

CLINICIAN: *OK. Now, let's see if you remember what we talked about last time. When do people usually feel sad, Lucas?*

LUCAS: *I think you said when you lose something.*

CLINICIAN: *Or someone. That's absolutely right. Sadness is the emotion we feel when we lose something or someone important to us. I know that you really didn't lose Leo in that situation because he was right there playing in your apartment. But, another way to see it is that you lost the chance to hang out and play with him. Does that make sense to you, Lucas?*

LUCAS: *I think so.*

ADRIANA: *That makes total sense to me! If Leo or Ana, his sister, doesn't want to play with him, he can get very sad. That's when he'll just disappear to his bedroom—when he really wants to be with them but can't.*

LUCAS: *I don't know why Leo and Ana don't want to play with me.*

ADRIANA: *They do want to play with you, Lucas, but not all the time. Sometimes they want to play with other people or just by themselves. You need to learn to be OK with that.*

CLINICIAN: *Exactly, Adriana! The way I see it, Lucas, is that in this situation, even though you wanted to play, you ended up not playing and hung out in your bedroom doing nothing instead. This situation is another example of a negative emotion, sadness, motivating you to go away or leave the situation and not do what you wanted—play and have fun. My guess is that this is also what's happening at school when certain classmates don't want to play with you, or you aren't asked to join them in some activity. Then, you end up feeling sad and not playing anything or with anyone during recess. So, my question to you, Lucas, is this. Do you want to learn how to handle and regulate your*

> *sadness so that you don't go to your bedroom and do nothing and be able to play instead?*
>
> Lucas: *Uh-huh.*
>
> Clinician: *That's great! I bet that if you can learn how to do this, you'll end up playing more during recess at school because you'll be able to handle or cope with your sadness there too.*
>
> Adriana: *I agree. That would be great!*

To review, here is what was covered in this part of the session:

- With the aid of the worksheet, the child was able to identify a situation that elicited a negative emotion, sadness, to a significant degree
- The parent was encouraged to add clarifying information, which included the child shutting down and not engaging in any productive behavior
- The clinician reminded the child and parent that sadness is an emotional reaction to a sense of loss
- The clinician described that sadness is another negative emotion that typically motivates people to act in ways to decrease the internal experience or to be removed from the source of emotional stimulation
- The clinician described how this experience was an episode of emotion dysregulation due to the intensity of the sadness and the resulting behavior
- The clinician confirmed that the parent wants the behavior to change, and that the child wants to learn how to effect this modification

At this point in the session, the clinician can continue reviewing and discussing other episodes documented on the worksheet. Using the protocol described above, reinforcing the learning of emotion identification skills with these two emotions is conducted. If the clinician decides to move on, then the following between-session activity is introduced and described.

> Clinician: *Before we move on to the last part of our meeting, I want to talk to you more about doing the emotion identification activity again this week. First, I want you, Lucas, to continue to complete rows on a new worksheet about situations that made you feel the emotions, "anger" or "sadness." Again, the more you practice, the better you'll get with this skill. However, I want to talk about another emotion for you to learn how to identify. The emotion is called "worry" or "feeling worried." Sometimes, people use the words, "nervous" or "anxious," which basically mean the same thing as worried. Do you ever feel worried, Lucas?*
>
> Lucas: *Is it the same as scared?*
>
> Clinician: *Feeling scared or worried is pretty similar but not quite the same thing. People feel worried or experience the emotion, "worry", when something bad or negative might happen in the future—the situation hasn't happened yet. When we feel scared or afraid—the emotion is*

called 'fear'—something bad or negative is happening right now or at the present time. Does that make sense?

ADRIANA: *I'm not sure. I've always thought that Lucas feels scared when he hears something loud, like his brother sometimes shouting when he plays video games.*

CLINICIAN: *Interesting point, Adriana. But, because nothing bad or negative is happening at the time, Lucas doesn't have anything to be scared of or fear. On the other hand, he might expect that something bad could still happen later on, and the related emotion in this situation is worry—also known as anxiety or nervousness.*

ADRIANA: *So, feeling scared is all about something bad now, and feeling worried is about the future.*

CLINICIAN: *That's right, Adriana. Now, let me say one more thing about the emotion, worry. The "something bad or negative" part is really about expecting some type of situation that might hurt or harm us in some way, such as getting physically injured or sick. For example, worry about getting COVID-19 has been an emotion that most of us have been feeling ever since the pandemic started. But, people can also feel worried about getting* emotionally *hurt or harmed. For you, Lucas, my guess is that you feel worried before every math quiz or test because you expect not to do very well. Is that true?*

LUCAS: *I think I'm going to get an "F" every time.*

CLINICIAN: *That thinking or thought you have is part of feeling worried. If you actually failed a math test, how would you feel emotionally?*

LUCAS: *I would be really upset.*

CLINICIAN: *That makes sense, Lucas, because pretty much everyone would feel that way if they failed a test. Feeling upset is one of those emotions that hurts or feels painful. Just like physical pain, emotional hurt or pain feels "bad on the inside." So, that's probably what your worry is all about with math quizzes or tests. You feel worried that you'll get a bad grade and feel upset. Does that sound right to you, Lucas?*

LUCAS: *I guess so.*

CLINICIAN: *Let's go back to what your mom said about you hearing loud sounds, like your brother yelling when playing video games. Do you think that his loud voice makes you feel worried?*

LUCAS: *Uh-huh.*

CLINICIAN: *Besides your brother, does anyone else in your family have a loud voice?*

LUCAS: *My dad.*

CLINICIAN: *When does he get loud?*

LUCAS: *When he drinks [alcohol].*

CLINICIAN: *Oh, OK. Then, do you feel the emotion, worry, when your dad's voice gets loud?*

LUCAS: *My dad can get really mean when he drinks* (Lucas nods his head "yes").

CLINICIAN: *How do you end up feeling emotionally when your dad's being mean to you?*

LUCAS: *Upset.*

CLINICIAN: *Again, feeling upset emotionally hurts or is painful. So, no wonder you feel worried when your dad gets loud. His loud voice is a sign or signal that you might become upset. Because we know that negative emotions can sometimes motivate people to leave situations that make them feel that way, my guess is that you go somewhere else in your apartment away from the loudness.*

ADRIANA: *Instead of just going to his bedroom and looking out the window, Lucas will crawl into bed, pull the covers over his head, and cry. He does this even when it's his brother who's being loud.*

LUCAS: Lucas looks down to avoid eye contact while his mother states the observation above.

CLINICIAN: *This situation is a great example of the ones that I want you to identify and write down on the next worksheet, Lucas. So, for this week, I want you to focus on three emotions—anger, sadness, and worry. Just like before, when you notice that you've felt one of these emotions, write down the name of the emotion in the middle part of the row. Then, work "backwards" and write down the situation that happened before you started feeling the emotion on the left side of the row. After that, write down how you acted or behaved on the right side. Do you have any questions, Lucas?*

LUCAS: *Nuh-uh.*

ADRIANA: *I do. Should I give him a reward like last time when he completes a row?*

CLINICIAN: *Absolutely. Also, if you notice that he experienced one of these emotions but didn't fill out the worksheet afterward, encourage him to do so. Of course, you can continue to help him fill out the worksheet if needed.*

ADRIANA: *Got it.*

To review, here is what was covered in this part of the session:

- The clinician introduced and described an additional negative emotion, worry, which is also known as anxiety or nervousness
- The clinician distinguished worry from fear
- A couple of situations that elicited worry were discussed
- The clinician described to the child and parent that worry is an emotional reaction to an expectation of being hurt, physically or emotionally

- The clinician requested that the child continue to conduct emotion identification training at home (with the addition of "worry" to "anger" and "sadness") by continuing to complete the Emotion Identification Worksheet

Introduction of emotion regulation skills. In this final part of the session, the clinician introduces emotion regulation training. The clinician begins by querying the child and parent to see if the child already possesses an activity in their repertoire that can be learned for use as an emotion regulation strategy, which is often the case. The central premise is that engaging in an activity that elicits internal positive emotions (i.e., happiness, satisfaction) will aid in decreasing the child's negative emotions. Activities that meet the following characteristics should be considered (in addition to their elicitation of positivity):

- Done independently
- Conducted for several minutes in duration uninterrupted (~10–15 minutes)
- Performed relatively quietly
- Carried out in a sedentary/seated position

If no activity meeting these criteria is present in the child's repertoire, a new activity will need to be identified. As long as they're developmentally appropriate and acceptable to the parent, as many activities as possible should be considered.

CLINICIAN: *So, here's when we start working to help you, Lucas, learn how to better cope with or regulate your emotions. As I've said before, the way that I want you to see this work is that you can learn how to make yourself feel better when you're feeling "emotionally bad" on the inside—that is, when you're experiencing a negative emotion, such as anger, sadness, or worry. With kids like you, the first thing that comes to my mind is that they usually feel good when playing with something. Is there a toy or game you play with that's really fun for you, Lucas?*

LUCAS: *I like playing video games.*

CLINICIAN: *I bet you do! But, I want to come up with something that will help you feel more calm and relaxed or "chill." Can you think of anything else?*

ADRIANA: *What about PLUS PLUS, Lucas?*

LUCAS: *Yeah. I like PLUS PLUS too.*

CLINICIAN: *What's PLUS PLUS? I've never heard of it.*

LUCAS: *They're blocks that you can build things with.*

CLINICIAN: *Interesting. Why are they called PLUS PLUS?*

ADRIANA: *Each block looks like two plus signs connected to each other. I think you get more than 200 blocks in each package.*

CLINICIAN: *What do you like to make with these blocks?*

LUCAS: *All sorts of things.*

CLINICIAN: *That's great! I have a couple of questions. First, do you play with PLUS PLUS by yourself or with your brother or sister?*

LUCAS: *Leo doesn't like playing with them anymore. Sometimes, I'll play with Ana but mostly by myself.*

CLINICIAN: *Got it. Next question—when you play PLUS PLUS, how long do you play before you stop or start playing something else?*

LUCAS: *I don't know.*

ADRIANA: *My best guess is that you play with those blocks for 15-20 minutes before you do something else.*

LUCAS: *Oh, OK.*

CLINICIAN: *So, it sounds like you can pay attention to those blocks and play with them for a pretty long time. My next question is for you, Adriana. Does Lucas play quietly with PLUS PLUS, or is he kind of loud?*

ADRIANA: *He's really quiet when he's making things with the blocks.*

CLINICIAN: *Perfect. Lucas, when you play with PLUS PLUS, do you play with them while sitting on the floor?*

LUCAS: *Uh-huh. I'll sometimes lie down on my tummy too.*

CLINICIAN: *Well, based on everything I've heard, I think that PLUS PLUS could be a great activity for you to learn to use for helping yourself handle or regulate your emotions. To do this well, you'll need to practice at home. This is what I want you to do. Adriana, whenever you have a chance this week to help Lucas in the afternoon before you start making dinner, I want you to see what Lucas is up to in your apartment. If you see that he is doing fine and not experiencing any negative emotions—meaning that he is well-regulated—I want you to go up to him and give him a verbal instruction, such as "Take a break," or another phrase that you two agree on. The most important part, Adriana, is that you use the same phrase or words for every practice opportunity. Lucas, when you hear those words, I want you to stop whatever you're doing, go to your bedroom or another room of your apartment where you can be by yourself, and play PLUS PLUS for 10 minutes. Adriana, if Lucas follows your instructions and starts playing with the blocks, I want you to set the timer on your mobile phone for 10 minutes and start the countdown with your phone on vibrate mode. When the timer goes off, I want you to check on Lucas to see that he's still playing with the blocks. Do either of you have any questions so far?*

LUCAS: *I just have to play PLUS PLUS for 10 minutes?*

CLINICIAN: *That's all you have to do, Lucas.*

ADRIANA: *What if Lucas doesn't listen to me and play with the blocks?*

CLINICIAN: *You just continue on with what you were doing before giving him the verbal instruction. Hopefully, Lucas will follow through every time for a few reasons. First, Lucas has said that he really wants to learn how to handle and regulate his emotions. Second, you'll be telling him to do something that he has fun doing and when he's in a well-regulated state, which means he'll be highly likely to listen to you. Third, I want you, Adriana, to reward him every time he does listen to you and play PLUS PLUS. Give him a reward just like you've done when he's completed a row on the Emotion Identification Worksheet.*

ADRIANA: *OK. Is that it?*

CLINICIAN: *Actually, two more things. Besides giving Lucas the verbal instruction, I also want you to give him a visual cue or sign at the same time. The cue can be something as simple as gently pulling on your left earlobe or swooping the front of your hair to one side. Again, you and Lucas can decide together what cue or sign is a good one to use. The reason for combining a visual cue with the verbal instruction is that with enough practice opportunities, the visual cue will become "equal" to the verbal instruction. When that happens, then, Adriana, you'll be able to use just the visual cue alone. As long as you can make eye contact with Lucas, giving him only the visual cue will be the same as "telling" him what he needs to do—play with PLUS PLUS to regulate his emotions or with other activities to be identified in the future that will also help him regulate.*

Ideally, I want you, Adriana, to practice with Lucas every day because "practice makes permanent." However, I know that you have a busy personal and family life, which I can understand because I've raised kids myself. So, if a day or a couple of days go by and you didn't get a chance to practice with Lucas, that's OK. I just want you to try your best and not worry at all if you don't practice every day.

Before we end today's meeting, I just want to say to you, Lucas, that my best guess is that you'll be able to learn this skill in regulating your emotions pretty easily as long as you practice and work at it. I also want to tell you that you don't need to come to the next couple of meetings because I only need to meet with your mom. As I see it, I'm your mom's coach—a parenting coach. She'll be able to tell me how your practicing at home has been going, and then I'll be able to give her tips or pointers on how you two can work together better so that your learning improves. Does that make sense, Lucas?

LUCAS: *Uh-huh.*

CLINICIAN: *Great! But, don't worry. We'll meet at least one more time before we end our work together. Adriana, I'll see you next week. Please remember to bring in the Emotion Identification Worksheet.*

Part II: Teaching Emotion Regulation Skills

The second part of TIP[s] is focused on training the parent to teach the child emotion regulation skills. Thus, treatment sessions include the parent only (except for the final one when the child is required to attend). This treatment modality targets a vital aspect of the family system whereby the parent's impact as an immediate extrinsic process is leveraged to facilitate and bolster the child's ability to regulate their emotions and related behavior. The approach to parent training is a stepwise one in which the parent is guided to teach their child emotion regulation by practicing skills across increasing intensity of emotion, specifically from none, to low, and lastly to a moderate level of intensity. Use of reinforcement is also bolstered to motivate the child to practice and to solidify their learning. The following script highlights how emotion regulation training initially unfolds.

Session 3 - Emotion Regulation Training

At the end of the session, the parent will be able to:

- Continue facilitating their child's improvement in emotion identification
- Begin the next step in between-session work of emotion regulation training in which the child will be prompted to engage in a regulating activity while experiencing emotions at a mild level of intensity

CLINICIAN: *Hi Adriana. Great to see you today. I'm wondering how Lucas did with learning how to identify his emotions this past week. Did you bring the Emotion Identification Worksheet?*

ADRIANA: *I completely forgot! But, I decided to take a picture of it with my mobile phone last night just in case* (a great idea indeed). *Lucas had a rough week. Whenever he sees his dad, he gets really irritable, and it takes a couple of days for him to calm down and get back to normal.*

CLINICIAN: *I see. So, did he fill out any rows of the worksheet?*

ADRIANA: *He did a few of them, but I had to remind him a lot. As you can see here* (Adriana unlocks her mobile phone and shows me the picture of the worksheet), *there were several times when Leo was pretty loud while playing video games, and Lucas became really nervous each time and crawled into his bed and cried. He also got angry a couple of times this week when I told him to finish his homework.*

CLINICIAN: *Did he end up leaving your apartment and going to the stairwell?*

ADRIANA: *He sure did!*

CLINICIAN: *Well, hopefully, he'll be able to learn to regulate his emotions soon so that he doesn't do that anymore. Does the worksheet indicate that he experienced sadness at all last week?*

ADRIANA: *A couple of times too. Just like before, it happened when Ana or Leo didn't want to play with him.*

CLINICIAN: *Did Lucas write down something about looking out his bedroom window when he was sad?*

ADRIANA: *For each row he completed.*

CLINICIAN: *It sounds like he did a great job again filling out the worksheet this week. How much did you reward or reinforce him for filling out the rows?*

ADRIANA: *Although I gave him a reward every time, Lucas actually reminded me a couple of times that I needed to reward him because he completed a row.*

CLINICIAN: *Good for you for reinforcing him, Adriana! I want to point out that I usually use the words, "reinforce" and "reinforcement," instead of "reward," especially with parents and other adults. I use those words because they specifically refer to increasing or improving positive behavior, not just giving something to kids afterward because they like it. One thing that I always tell parents is that they need to reinforce good/positive/acceptable/appropriate behavior just as much as or more than punishing bad/negative/unacceptable/inappropriate behavior. Although I usually don't have to teach parents how to punish negative behavior, I often have to remind, if not teach, them how to reinforce positive behavior.*

At this point, how well do you think Lucas can identify feeling angry, sad, and anxious/worried?

ADRIANA: *I'm surprised how good he's getting at it! He's picked it up pretty fast.*

CLINICIAN: *That's awesome! To make sure he gets quite good at identifying his emotions, I want him to continue this work at home by completing another worksheet and for you to continue helping and reminding him when needed. Are you OK with that, Adriana?*

ADRIANA: *Absolutely!*

CLINICIAN: *Although anger, sadness, and anxiety seem to be the main negative emotions Lucas struggles with, we can also have Lucas learn to identify other ones too, especially if he starts to have problems with them in the future. Two of these emotions are closely related, "guilt" and "shame." Both are associated with wrongdoing or being wrong. The difference is that feeling guilty is associated with our alleged "wrong" behavior, and feeling ashamed is related to perceiving ourselves as "wrong" in a fundamental way as a whole person. In other words, guilt is about our actions, and shame is our being as humans. Does that make sense, Adriana?*

ADRIANA: *I think so. I'm now wondering if Lucas feels ashamed of himself because he always says, "I'm stupid," whenever we talk about how he's doing in school. Unfortunately, his father would call him "stupid"* and "lazy" when Lucas would ask him for help with his homework. This would happen a lot when his father was drunk, and Lucas would end up shutting down and crying in his bed.

CLINICIAN: *I really appreciate you sharing that information, Adriana. Based on those situations with his father, which is a form of emotional abuse, I wouldn't be surprised at all that Lucas experiences the emotion of shame, especially when it comes to his identity as a student. At this point, I'll leave things up to you about introducing shame to Lucas's work in learning to identify his emotions.*

To review, here is what was covered in this first part of the session:

- The clinician confirmed that the child completed the emotion identification activity and associated worksheet
- With the aid of the worksheet, the parent was able to review several situations that elicited the child's negative emotions, which the child documented on the worksheet
- The clinician praised the parent for reinforcing the child's practice at home and encouraged her to continue doing so
- The clinician requested that the child continue with the emotion identification work and for the parent's ongoing assistance and guidance
- The clinician introduced the option of adding other emotions for the child to learn to identify, specifically shame and guilt

CLINICIAN: *So, let's now talk about the emotion regulation work. Were you able to practice with Lucas using the PLUS PLUS blocks as a regulation activity?*

ADRIANA: *I was able to do it about 3-4 times this week.*

CLINICIAN: *How did things go?*

ADRIANA: *Surprisingly well! We used your suggestion, "Take a break," as the words to tell him what to do. I also came up with the idea of tucking my hair behind my left ear as the visual cue, which Lucas agreed to.*

CLINICIAN: *That's great. How well did he follow through and play with the blocks for 10 minutes?*

ADRIANA: *He did it every single time! One thing that really helped is that I remembered that he likes to stay up later on the weekends and play video games with his brother. So, I told him that he could stay up 15 minutes longer on school nights to play video games whenever he listened to me and played PLUS PLUS.*

CLINICIAN: *What a brilliant way to reinforce him for practicing! I'm quite impressed with you, Adriana.*

ADRIANA: *Thanks!*

CLINICIAN: *At this point, how well do you think that Lucas has learned this procedure?*

ADRIANA: *Very well. But, it was easy for him because we practiced when he was in a good mood, just like you told us to do.*

CLINICIAN: *That's right. I precisely had you practice this way because learning is best, at least initially, when we're in a calm and relaxed state and not stressed out. Besides you doing a wonderful job reinforcing him, this is probably another reason that Lucas learned the process quickly. Also, because he already knew how to play with the blocks, he didn't have to learn something new, which likely was helpful too. He just learned to play with PLUS PLUS under different conditions—when you tell him to instead of when he wants to.*

However, we now need to go to the next step, which is that Lucas needs to learn to play with the blocks as a regulation activity when he's actually experiencing one of the negative emotions that he struggles with. Here's what I want you to do. Instead of looking for and practicing with Lucas when he's well-regulated and in a good mood, I want you to try your best to "catch him" when something's happened, and he's experiencing a negative emotion. For example, I can imagine that sometimes he might feel angry when doing homework because he's confused about what to do. If you see him in a situation like that and the intensity of his anger seems low, not medium or high, that's when I want you to give him the verbal instruction, "Take a break," and the visual cue you came up with. The main indicator that a negative emotion is at a low level of intensity is that his behavior is in line with what you expect him to be doing at that time—in this case, continuing on with his homework. The idea here is that if his negative emotion isn't overwhelming him to the point where he feels out of control, he should be able to hear your instruction, see your visual cue, and decide to play with PLUS PLUS. How does that sound to you, Adriana?

ADRIANA: *I think I get it. But, what do I do when I notice that his negative emotion is at a medium or high level?*

CLINICIAN: *That's a great question. I appreciate you for asking it. In that case, I don't want you to practice with Lucas. Just do what you normally would do, which makes me want to ask, "What would that be?"*

ADRIANA: *I usually talk to him and ask him what's wrong. If he's really upset, I hold him and give him a hug.*

CLINICIAN: *Does that usually work?*

ADRIANA: *It does, but it can take a few minutes before he calms down.*

CLINICIAN: *Well, it definitely seems like you have a calming presence for him, which is great. So, keep doing what you've been doing if the intensity of his emotion is at a medium or high level. From Lucas's point of view, the practicing should be the same as before. Whenever he hears the verbal instruction and sees the visual cue, he just has to stop what he's doing and go play with the blocks for 10 minutes. However, from your perspective, there'll be one difference—you'll be instructing and cueing him when he's experiencing a low level of negative emotion rather than when he's well-regulated and fully engaged in an activity. Just like last time, set your phone timer for 10 minutes and give him a reinforcer when you confirm after the vibrator goes off that he's been playing with PLUS PLUS. Before we end our meeting today, I'm wondering if you can think of a situation that would make Lucas feel a little sad or anxious?*

ADRIANA: *He gets a bit worried whenever he hears me talking to his dad on the phone.*

CLINICIAN: *I can fully understand that emotional reaction given the types of experiences he's had with his father. That situation might be a really good one for you to try to give him just the visual cue alone because you'll be on the phone. What do you think?*

ADRIANA: *It makes perfect sense to me.*

CLINICIAN: *Well, best of luck with the practicing this week. I'm confident that you and Lucas will do great!*

To review, here is what was covered in the final part of the session:

- The clinician confirmed that the parent conducted the emotion regulation practice with the child
- The clinician verified that the parent used both a verbal instruction and visual cue to prompt the child to engage with the identified regulation activity
- The clinician confirmed that the parent reinforced the child's practicing and praised them for doing so
- The clinician introduced the next step of between-session work of emotion regulation training in which the child will be prompted to engage in a regulating activity while experiencing a negative emotion of low intensity

Session 4 - Emotion Regulation Training

At the end of the session, the parent will be able to:

- Continue facilitating their child's improvement in emotion identification (if needed)
- Begin the next step of between-session work of emotion regulation training when the child is experiencing emotions at a moderate level of intensity

CLINICIAN: *Hi Adriana. I hope you, Lucas, and your other kids had a good week. Overall, how was Lucas since we last met?*

ADRIANA: *Pretty good, I guess. But, I did get an email from his teacher, who said that Lucas is still not playing with his classmates during recess and just sits around doing nothing.*

CLINICIAN: *Thanks for letting me know about his behavior at recess. As we've talked about before, that reaction is probably very similar to the sadness he experiences when his brother or sister doesn't want to play with him. Hopefully, when he learns to better regulate his emotions at home, he'll also be able to do so at school, which means that the chances of him playing with classmates will increase. How did he do with the emotion identification practice?*

ADRIANA: *Really, really well! In fact, he continued to remind me when I forgot to reward, I mean reinforce, him for completing a row on the worksheet. He's gotten pretty good at knowing when he feels angry, sad, and anxious.*

CLINICIAN: *How great is that?! I'm quite proud of Lucas and hope you are too.*

ADRIANA: *Definitely! And I know he's also proud of himself because he really likes to show me completed rows on the worksheet.*

CLINICIAN: *And don't forget about your efforts, Adriana. You're the one who's kept him on track with the practice and reinforced him for doing the work. If it weren't for you, he probably wouldn't have learned as much as he has. So congratulations are in order for a job well done.*

ADRIANA: *Thanks so much.*

CLINICIAN: *So, let's put that practicing on hold for now, given how good he's gotten at identifying his anger, sadness, and anxiety. Like I mentioned last time, we can work on Lucas identifying other emotions, such as shame and guilt, if he starts having problems with them in the future. In the meantime, we'll focus on his emotion regulation. How did things go in getting him to play PLUS PLUS when his emotion was at a low level of intensity?*

ADRIANA: *It actually was pretty hard. I guess I didn't realize that his emotions can sometimes be not so intense because I'm usually not paying attention to him until he gets very upset. So, it took me a little while to notice when his emotions were mild.*

CLINICIAN: *Can you share an example with me?*

ADRIANA: *One night, Lucas was kind of distracted and slowly eating his dinner. His sister and brother finished before him, and he didn't realize he was the last one to finish eating until his brother turned on the TV and videogame. Then, because he wanted to play with Leo, he quickly ate the rest of his dinner. However, I told him that he needed to help me put the dirty dishes in the sink before he could go play. That's when he got a little angry at me.*

CLINICIAN: *Did you tell him, "Take a break," and give him the visual cue?*

ADRIANA: *Just the visual cue. And he actually went to play PLUS PLUS right away for 10 minutes.*

CLINICIAN: *That's great! And did you reinforce him for following through?*

ADRIANA: *I sure did. I let him play video games for an extra 15 minutes before getting ready for bed.*

CLINICIAN: *Good for you, Adriana! Does another example come to mind?*

ADRIANA: *Sometime last weekend, Lucas was watching TV with Leo and Ana. I noticed that after a while, Lucas was getting bored and wanted to watch something else. But, Leo wanted to continue watching the show and told Lucas that he could leave if he didn't want to watch that show. I then saw that Lucas had a sad look on his face. So, I went up to him and told him, Take a break."*

CLINICIAN: *Did he go and play with the blocks again?*

ADRIANA: *Not this time. Although I told him, "Remember what you're working for," he said that he wanted to continue watching TV.*

CLINICIAN: *What did you end up doing?*

ADRIANA: *I tucked my hair behind my left ear to see if that cue would work, but it didn't. So, I just left him alone to be with Leo and Ana.*

CLINICIAN: *That's perfect! The way that I want you to understand this practicing is that when you verbally or visually prompt Lucas to play with the blocks, you're letting him know that he has the opportunity to help himself feel better emotionally. However, Lucas is the one who's responsible for deciding whether or not to engage in the regulating activity. In other words, you can't "make him" relax or calm down. He has to choose to do so and put in the effort to feel better. You're actually teaching him to take control of himself in situations that are emotionally challenging for him. How many times do you remember practicing with him this week?*

ADRIANA: *I think five times.*

CLINICIAN: *And how many times did Lucas follow through and play PLUS PLUS?*

ADRIANA: *I remember that he didn't play with the blocks one time. So, he played with them four times.*

CLINICIAN: *Well, four out of five times is 80%, which is a very good percentage. At this point, how confident are you that Lucas can now regulate his emotions when they're at a low level of intensity?*

ADRIANA: *Fairly confident, but I want to be very confident that he can do it.*

CLINICIAN: *Me too. So, let's have you continue practicing with Lucas the same way you've been doing, although you can probably stop using the verbal instruction and just use the visual cue. Also, continue reinforcing him when he follows through and plays PLUS PLUS. Keep up the practice until your confidence is quite high that Lucas can regulate his emotions at low-intensity levels by playing with the blocks. You don't need to have complete or 100% confidence. If your confidence level is at 80% or more, that should be good enough. Agreed?*

ADRIANA: *Agreed. What happens after that?*

CLINICIAN: *The next step is for you to cue Lucas when you notice that he's experiencing a negative emotion at a moderate level of intensity. My understanding is that Lucas really struggles when his emotions are moderately intense. Based on my clinical experience, this step is the hardest one to practice because emotions at that level begin to interfere with a person's ability to stay engaged with the situation or activity at hand. In other words, they start to lose emotional control and behave in unhelpful ways. Can you think of a situation that leads to Lucas feeling moderately angry, sad, or anxious?*

ADRIANA: *When his brother or sister doesn't want to play with him, I think his sadness is usually at that level. And that's when he'll go to his bedroom and stare out the window.*

CLINICIAN: *That makes sense to me, which is why that situation will be a great one to work on with him. For the practicing to be most effective, I want you to try your best to cue Lucas as soon as you realize that Leo or Ana has refused to play with him. Another reason that this step is the hardest one to work on is that you're going to have to pay close attention so that you can cue him right after he starts experiencing the emotion. If you cue him early enough, Lucas will hopefully decide to start playing with the blocks before he has a chance to behave in unhelpful ways, such as staring out the window. That's the goal.*

ADRIANA: *That would be amazing if he could learn to do that!*

CLINICIAN: *Now, what about his anger? When can he be moderately angry?*

ADRIANA: *I'm not sure.*

CLINICIAN: *You've mentioned that he can get a little angry doing homework. Does his homework ever lead him to be even angrier?*

ADRIANA: *You're right about asking that. In his mind, if he has a lot of math homework or thinks that it will take a long time to finish it, he can get pretty angry.*

CLINICIAN: *Does he do or say anything that lets you know that his anger is at that level?*

ADRIANA: *When he says, "I hate math," that's when I know.*

CLINICIAN: *So, in that situation, do your best to cue him as soon as those words come out of his mouth.*

ADRIANA: *Got it!*

CLINICIAN: *Like before, if Lucas doesn't follow through and play PLUS PLUS, do what you normally would do in those situations. Also, reinforce him if he does play with the blocks after you cue him. Because this step is the hardest one, I encourage you to give him bigger or more reinforcers when he follows through. For example, instead of 15 minutes, let him stay up to play for 20 minutes before he has to get ready for bed. Do you have any questions before we end today's meeting?*

ADRIANA: *Not really.*

CLINICIAN: *Then, please give my best to Lucas, and good luck with practicing this week.*

To review, here is what was covered in the session:

- The clinician assessed and ascertained from the parent's report that the child continued to exhibit problems at school
- The clinician confirmed that the child continued to work on identifying emotions
- The clinician reinforced the parent's effort in facilitating their child's practice with emotion identification
- The clinician and parent jointly agreed that the child's skill in identifying emotions is at an adequate level of performance
- The clinician verified that the parent conducted the emotion regulation practice with the child while the emotions were at a mild level of intensity
- The clinician confirmed that the parent reinforced the child's practicing and praised them for doing so
- The clinician and parent jointly agreed that the child needs more practice at this step in which their emotions are mildly intense
- The clinician instructed the parent to drop the verbal instruction and just use the visual cue
- The clinician instructed the parent to continue with this step until they are very confident in their child's skill at regulating emotions at a mild level
- The clinician introduced the next step of between-session work of emotion regulation training in which the child will be prompted to engage in a regulating activity while experiencing a negative emotion of moderate intensity

Session 5 - Emotion Regulation Training & Cognitive Restructuring

At the end of the session, the parent will be able to:

- Continue between-session work of emotion regulation training when the child is experiencing emotions at a moderate level of intensity
- Articulate the foundation and guiding principle of cognitive restructuring

CLINICIAN: *Hi Adriana. I hope you're doing well. How did Lucas's week go?*

ADRIANA: *He had a pretty good week, I think. But the practicing was hard for him.*

CLINICIAN: *How so?*

ADRIANA: *I decided to move to the next step just a couple of days after our last meeting because he was doing great with the practicing. But he didn't follow through very much with playing PLUS PLUS after that.*

CLINICIAN: *I'm not too surprised. How often do you think he played with the blocks when you cued him?*

ADRIANA: *About half the time.*

CLINICIAN: *It's challenging to make good decisions when our emotions are relatively intense. Because adults also have trouble making appropriate choices when they're experiencing a moderately intense emotion, we should expect that children will struggle even more when they're in that emotional state. Lucas's brain is clearly less developed than yours or mine, given his age, which means that he will need significant practice to learn to regulate his emotions when the intensity is that high. Of course, you will also need to put in a good amount of time and effort to facilitate his learning. How much are you willing to continue to do so, Adriana?*

ADRIANA: *As much as it takes. I love him so much, and I don't want him to continue to get so upset.*

CLINICIAN: *I'm pleased to know that. Given his current level of progress, I think it makes sense for you to continue with this step by cueing him when his emotion is moderately intense. Are you OK with that?*

ADRIANA: *Yes, I am.*

CLINICIAN: *How much practicing did you end up doing this past week?*

ADRIANA: *The practice didn't happen as much as the last step because there weren't many times when his emotions were at that intensity. But, there were definitely times when Lucas's emotions were really intense.*

CLINICIAN: *Can you give me an example?*

ADRIANA: *Although he's getting better because I keep telling him to be quiet, Leo sometimes will shout really loudly when something happens in the video game he's playing. If Lucas is close by, he will immediately go to his room and crawl into bed. That's a situation where he didn't follow through and play with the blocks.*

CLINICIAN: *I understand. To help make sure that Lucas doesn't take a step back in helping himself to feel better emotionally, let's also have you practice with him when his emotions are mildly intense. Just a couple of times a week should do it. But is there another game or toy he plays with that he likes just as much as PLUS PLUS? It's always good to have a couple of options when kids need to actively regulate their emotions.*

It also gives them a sense of being in control when they can choose for themselves instead of someone telling them what to do.

ADRIANA: *I'm not sure.*

CLINICIAN: *As a reminder, the activity needs to have these characteristics. First, the activity should be fun and rewarding—in other words, trigger positive emotions in Lucas. Second, the activity should be one that he usually plays by himself. Third, the activity needs to be interesting enough that Lucas can pay attention to and play with for about 10 minutes in a row without being distracted by anything else. Fourth, the activity should be designed to be played quietly. Lastly, the activity is best played in a seated position.*

ADRIANA: *I don't think Lucas plays with anything else that has all those things you just said.*

CLINICIAN: *Then, we need to find a new activity that he can learn to use as a regulating activity. I have two ideas. One is to download on your mobile phone a free app that's made for kids to help them calm down and relax. One of these apps is called "Stop, Breathe & Think Kids." Because Lucas likes to build things, another idea I have is to get some kinetic sand. This "sand" isn't real sand because it's made to stick only to itself, which means that it's not really messy. Lucas can mold the sand into any shape and build just about anything. My understanding is that it's relatively inexpensive. What do you think about these ideas?*

ADRIANA: *I like them both! Because Lucas likes playing video games, he might like the app. And the kinetic sand sounds really different, which he might like too. I'll download the app right away and see where I can buy the sand for a good price.*

CLINICIAN: *That's great! For the practicing, here's what I want you to say to Lucas. Tell him that you have a surprise for him to use to regulate his emotions, but don't tell him what they are. This week, when you first catch him experiencing a mild-intensity emotion, grab the sand and your mobile phone (open the app) before you go and give him the visual cue. Once you cue him, present both items and let him choose which one he wants. As always, he has to play with the item to help himself feel better emotionally. With a little bit of luck, he'll learn to use both of them as regulating activities. How does all this sound to you, Adriana?*

ADRIANA: *I'm excited to see if he'll like these activities. But what about practicing with the moderate-intensity emotions?*

CLINICIAN: *Hopefully, the addition of these new activities will increase the chance that he will choose to help himself feel better emotionally even when his emotions are moderately intense. As I said earlier, having a few options to choose from should increase his sense of being in control instead of him feeling that you're telling him what to do.*

ADRIANA: *I get it.*

CLINICIAN: *Another important point to all of this is that Lucas needs to be able to regulate his emotions in situations and settings beyond your apartment, such as in school. If he can use building or making things at home to help calm himself down, then he should be able to use similar materials or activities in his classroom to do the same. His teacher just needs to be told how Lucas has learned to use blocks, for example, as a way to regulate himself when he's experiencing negative emotions of significant intensity. They also need to be open to giving him permission and the opportunity to engage in a regulating activity in the classroom by using the visual cue just like you've learned how to do. If he has a hard time emotionally in different areas of the school, I'm hopeful that if he uses the mobile phone app enough times at home, he'll be able to use the skills at school even without the app, such as on the playground. How much do you think Lucas's teacher will be onboard if you tell them about his practicing and developing the ability to regulate his emotions?*

ADRIANA: *Because his teacher is great and seems to care about Lucas, I bet that they will be very interested in learning how Lucas has learned to cope with his emotions at home.*

CLINICIAN: *Then, I recommend that you reach out to them and let them know about Lucas's work and practicing. If you want, I can also contact them about it.*

To review, here is what was covered in the first part of the session:

- The clinician verified from the parent's report that they began the next step of emotion regulation training in which the child experiences emotions of moderate intensity
- The clinician assessed and ascertained from the parent's report that the child was only partially successful with the practicing
- The clinician described how moderately intense emotions are challenging to regulate for adults, let alone children
- The clinician and parent jointly agreed that continued practice with moderately intense emotions is required
- The clinician also recommended conducting some emotion regulation practice with emotions at a mild level of intensity to maintain the skill at an adequate performance level
- The clinician recommended identifying and introducing one or two new regulating activities in the practicing
- The clinician reviewed the essential characteristics of a regulating activity
- The clinician described how the child's developing skill in emotion regulation can be generalized to the school setting by informing the child's teacher about the work and learning that the child has accomplished at home

To end the session, the clinician introduces the cognitive component of emotions. The discussion is primarily psychoeducational and should initially focus on the child's likely cognitions as part of their emotional experiences. Then, the focus of the conversation should shift to the parent to begin to better understand their own emotions and associated cognitions. The goals of this exchange are twofold: (a) with help from the parent, the child learns to identify and alter the cognitive aspects of their emotions, and (b) the parent learns to identify and alter their own emotion-related cognitions. In essence, both goals are also enhanced emotion regulation but emphasize impacting cognitive factors. Known generically as cognitive restructuring or specifically as reappraisal, the overarching process involves intentionally changing how we think about and describe the meaning attributed to a stimulus and its source to alter our emotional reaction to that activity, event, or situation (Gross, 1998).

CLINICIAN: *Before we finish today's meeting, Adriana, I want to talk to you about another important aspect of emotions. The formal term is "cognition." However, the word that most everybody knows and basically means the same thing is "thoughts." Even though people usually view emotions and thoughts as different things that are experienced, what I want you to know is that emotions have cognitive components to them. In other words, emotions include thoughts. What this means is that what we think - our thoughts - and how we think - our thought processes - are part of our emotional experiences. Does that make sense?*

ADRIANA: *I'm not sure.*

CLINICIAN: *Let me give you an example. One important thing I learned from Lucas is that his anger can be triggered by schoolwork, especially math. He also shared his dislike of math when he said in one of our meetings, "I hate math."*

ADRIANA: *And he says that to me all the time.*

CLINICIAN: *So, when he says the words, "I hate math," he's basically letting us know that he has that thought or similar ones as part of his anger that's triggered by math. Does that make sense now?*

ADRIANA: *It sure does.*

CLINICIAN: *Great! Does anything else he says come to mind when he feels angry about math?*

ADRIANA: *Let me think. Yeah. He sometimes says, "Math is stupid."*

CLINICIAN: *That's a great example of another thought he probably has that's part of his math-related anger. Let's switch to another emotion, sadness. What has he said out loud when he feels sad?*

ADRIANA: *If his brother or sister doesn't want to play with him, he'll say either "Leo doesn't like me" or "Ana doesn't like me."*

CLINICIAN: *Given what we know about sadness, I can understand why he says those things. As a reminder, sadness is all about a sense of loss. In this case, he loses the opportunity to hang out and play with Leo or Ana when they don't want to play with him. He then probably thinks that they don't like him, which is part of the sadness that he feels.*

ADRIANA: And that's totally wrong. Leo and Ana love Lucas so much. They just sometimes don't want to play with him for reasons that don't have anything to do with him.

CLINICIAN: That I can understand. Unfortunately, if he continues to have these negative thoughts as part of his emotions, regulating his emotions will remain challenging for him. Moving forward, another way that you can help him then is to get him to identify his negative thoughts and change them to be more positive or at least less negative. For Lucas to understand what thoughts are, you might want to use the term, "self-talk," which is another way to label what he says to himself in silence, not out loud. Another way to put it is that thinking is simply "talking to yourself." Does all this make sense to you, Adriana?

ADRIANA: I like the words, "self-talk," and I think Lucas will understand what they mean.

CLINICIAN: That's great! Now, to help him learn to change his negative thoughts, I want you both to memorize the question, "What's the positive opposite?" A good time to ask him this question is when he's experiencing a negative emotion at a mild-intensity level, and he says something that tips you off about the cognitive component of the emotion, such as "Ana doesn't like me." When you hear negative words like that from Lucas, I want you to say something like this to him.

"I hear what you're saying, Lucas. But, I wonder if that's your sadness talking. My guess is that you wouldn't say that if you weren't feeling sad. Maybe you might feel better emotionally if you say something else that's more positive. [Clinician's name] told me an easy way to do this, which is to ask yourself the question, "What's the positive opposite?" Let me ask you now, Lucas, what's the positive opposite of "Ana doesn't like me"?"

To make sure you understand the point, Adriana, please tell me how Lucas should answer that question.

ADRIANA: He should say, "Ana likes me."

CLINICIAN: That's absolutely correct! From there, I would want you to say something like this to him.

You're right, Lucas. "Ana likes me" is the positive opposite of "Ana doesn't like me." If you want to feel less sad, you need to say that to yourself instead. [Clinician's name] told me that they sometimes call this "self-talk" or talking to yourself. Another reason to change your negative self-talk is that it really isn't true. I know how much Ana loves you and likes doing things with you. So, saying to yourself, "Ana doesn't like me," is wrong. "Ana likes me" is the right thing to say to yourself, or positive self-talk.

ADRIANA: *I think I can do that. But, what if he doesn't understand what to say or says the wrong thing?*

CLINICIAN: *Then, just give him the answer and explain what opposites are. My guess is that if you tell him a few opposite pairs, such as black-white, right-left, and up-down, he'll understand the meaning of "opposite" pretty quickly.*

ADRIANA: *Got it.*

CLINICIAN: *One more thing. Sometimes, the positive opposite thought is too extreme, which means that Lucas probably won't be OK with it because it's not true either. Here's a perfect example. Tell me, Adriana, what's the positive opposite of "I hate math?"*

ADRIANA: *"I love math." You're absolutely right. There's no way he'd be OK with saying "I love math" to himself.*

CLINICIAN: *Agreed. So, you would then ask him to come up with another phrase that's more positive but that he likes more. For example, "Math is OK" is a thought that probably would be more acceptable to him and one that's clearly more positive than "I hate math." Do you think I'm right?*

ADRIANA: *Yes. I think that Lucas could eventually learn to say "Math is OK" to himself.*

CLINICIAN: *Good to know. Again, the goal is that he will be able to identify his negative cognitions/thoughts/self-talk and replace them with more positive, or at least less negative, ones. Using the question, "What's the positive opposite?" is a great first step in getting kids as well as teens and adults to come up with healthier thoughts. With enough practice, Lucas should come to understand what this process is all about, even if the positive opposite question doesn't quite fit the situation. The expectation is that he'll learn to realize that his negative self-talk can be changed in positive ways that will also help in regulating his emotions.*

Because this strategy can also be useful for adults, I'm wondering, Adriana, what your thoughts are about using it for yourself.

ADRIANA: *I think it could be helpful for me too.*

CLINICIAN: *How so?*

ADRIANA: *I sometimes get pretty upset. After talking with you about negative thoughts and how they're part of our emotions, I now have a better idea of how my moods and emotions affect me.*

CLINICIAN: *I appreciate you for telling me that, Adriana. Can you give me an example?*

ADRIANA: *When Lucas gets very angry, and I can't calm him down, that's when I can get upset.*

CLINICIAN: *In those situations, I'm wondering what your negative cognitions are.*

ADRIANA: *One thing that I say to myself is, "You're such a lousy mother."*

CLINICIAN: *So, what's the positive opposite of that negative thought?*

ADRIANA: *"You're not a lousy mother."*

CLINICIAN: *Or "You're a good mother."*

ADRIANA: *I guess so.*

CLINICIAN: *To continue with this strategy of identifying and changing negative cognitions, the next step is to come up with evidence or facts to support the new thought. What comes to mind to help prove that you really are a good mother?*

ADRIANA: *Well, I've been taking care of my kids all by myself for several months now.*

CLINICIAN: *I do hope, Adriana, that you being a single parent raising three great kids does show you how good a mother you are. Also, I bet that there's not much evidence to support the idea that you're a lousy mother.*

ADRIANA: *I guess you're right.*

CLINICIAN: *So, if there's lots of evidence for the positive cognitions compared to the negative thoughts, it should make sense to go with and believe the positive ones. If you can do that, then you will have learned how you can better regulate your emotions by changing the cognitive components of them. You can also do this next step with Lucas. See if he can come up with "facts" to support his positive self-talk compared to his negative self-talk. If he can't do it, you can then give him a couple of examples to get him started, such as reminding him of something that Ana recently did that indicates that she really does like him rather than hate him. Before we end today's meeting, do you have any last questions?*

ADRIANA: *I don't think so.*

CLINICIAN: *Best of luck then as you continue to work and practice with Lucas on improving his skills in regulating his emotions.*

ADRIANA: *Thanks!*

To review, here is what was covered in the last part of the session:

- The clinician described how emotions have cognitive components
- A couple of examples of emotions were discussed to illustrate their cognitive components
- The clinician introduced the term, self-talk, as a developmentally appropriate alternative to the word, thought
- The clinician discussed how changing negative cognitions to positive (or less negative) ones is another means to regulate emotions
- The clinician introduced the question, *"What's the positive opposite?"*, as a tool to help identify positive cognitions

- The clinician described how the parent could help their child identify negative self-talk and use the positive opposite question to help them change negative cognitions to positive ones
- The clinician discussed how the parent could respond when the child has difficulty coming up with positive cognitions
- The clinician emphasized how the parent can use cognitive reappraisal to regulate their own emotions better
- The clinician discussed with the parent how such reappraising could be effected
- The clinician noted how evidence could be gathered and used to support positive cognitions

Session 6 - Emotion Regulation Training & Cognitive Restructuring

At the end of the session, the parent will be able to:

- Continue between-session work of emotion regulation training with their child
- Continue between-session work of cognitive restructuring with their child and themselves

CLINICIAN: *Hi Adriana. It's nice to see you again. Let's get right into it. Last week, we talked about you continuing to practice with Lucas when his emotions are at a moderate level of intensity. We also discussed identifying new regulating activities for him to use as well as doing some practicing when mild-intensity emotions are occurring so that he maintains his skills. We ended our meeting talking about negative cognitions or self-talk and how they can be identified and changed as an additional way to regulate emotions for both Lucas and you.*

ADRIANA: *Yeah. We talked about a lot last time. But, the practicing went much better this week.*

CLINICIAN: *That's great! Tell me more.*

ADRIANA: *For one thing, he followed through more when I cued him. I remember one situation where I heard Lucas say really loudly, "Why not, Ana?" after she said that she didn't want to play with him. I immediately went over to him and tucked my hair behind my ear. At first, he just stared at me with a sad look in his eyes. But then, he ended up going to his room and playing with the sand.*

CLINICIAN: *Oh! You got some kinetic sand.*

ADRIANA: *I did. I asked one of my friends who lives in the same apartment complex as me if she knew anything about the sand. She told me exactly where to go to buy it.*

CLINICIAN: *That's awesome! And what's even better is that Lucas was able to use the sand to regulate himself.*

ADRIANA: *I know! He even followed through one time when he was pretty mad because of a math assignment he was doing.*

CLINICIAN: *I'm so proud of Lucas and you too, Adriana. It sounds like your work with him is paying off. What about mild-intensity emotions? Did you do any practicing with those?*

ADRIANA: *That's how I introduced the kinetic sand to him. After I bought it, I showed him the sand right after cueing him one time when he looked like he was getting anxious because I raised my voice at Leo when he wasn't listening to me. As soon as he saw it, he grabbed it from my hand, went to his room, and played with it.*

CLINICIAN: *So, he's using the sand as a regulating activity just like PLUS PLUS, correct?*

ADRIANA: *That's right.*

CLINICIAN: *Again, awesome! Did you also introduce a relaxation app?*

ADRIANA: *I downloaded the app you mentioned last week to my phone. But I haven't shown it to Lucas yet. Because he did so great with the sand right away, I decided to hold off on the app.*

CLINICIAN: *Your decision seems like an excellent one given how well he's now using the sand as a regulating activity in addition to the blocks. At this point, how confident are you that Lucas can regulate his emotions at mild- or moderate-intensity levels?*

ADRIANA: *I'm very confident. But I think he could use a little more practice just to be completely sure.*

CLINICIAN: *I like your thinking, Adriana. Go ahead then and continue practicing with him this week. At this point, practice when his emotions are either mildly or moderately intense. This will also give you a chance to introduce the app as another activity for him to learn to use to regulate his emotions. As I said last week, having a few options to choose from should increase his sense of being in control instead of him feeling that you're telling him what to do.*

ADRIANA: *Got it.*

CLINICIAN: *Moving on, did you talk to Lucas about self-talk and that cognitions or thoughts are part of our emotional experiences?*

ADRIANA: *I decided to bring it up one time when we were talking about school the other day and he said to me, "I have no friends."*

CLINICIAN: *What did you say to him?*

ADRIANA: *I took your advice and told him that was his sadness talking and that emotions include talking to ourselves or self-talk. I then asked him the opposite question.*

CLINICIAN: *You mean the positive opposite question?*

ADRIANA: *I'm sorry. Yes. The positive opposite question.*

CLINICIAN: *Was he able to come up with a positive cognition?*

ADRIANA: *Not right away. I had to tell him that the positive opposite of "I have no friends" is "I have friends."*

CLINICIAN: *Good for you, Adriana! What happened after that?*

ADRIANA: *I told him that he does have friends and reminded him of his friend, Jack, who's the son of my friend who told me where to get the kinetic sand.*

CLINICIAN: *You did a great job introducing self-talk to Lucas. Was that the only time you talked about cognitions with him?*

ADRIANA: *There was one more time when he said that Leo doesn't like him. And he was able to say, "Leo likes me," when I asked him the positive opposite question. I then told Lucas that sometimes he has to be patient with Leo when he doesn't want to play with him and that it doesn't mean that Leo doesn't like him just because he says "No."*

CLINICIAN: *Terrific again, Adriana. Did you also explain to him that changing his negative self-talk to positive self-talk is another way to regulate his emotions or to make himself feel better emotionally?*

ADRIANA: *I did. But I don't think he gets it yet.*

CLINICIAN: *That's OK. You're on the right track. He just needs more practice with it. To help him better understand and learn the concept of cognitions or self-talk, you two can use the Emotion Identification Worksheet together as a guide. Besides writing down the name of the emotion in the middle part of each row, he can also write his negative self-talk in those sections. If you kept any of the old worksheets, you can go back to them and ask Lucas to think about possible cognitions he had as part of the emotion he experienced at the time. Whether reviewing old worksheets or working on new ones, your job, Adriana, is to ask him the positive opposite question for each thought that's written on them. Just like before, verbally praise him in the moment when he's working with you and reinforce him for his efforts.*

ADRIANA: *Those are great suggestions.*

CLINICIAN: *What about you, Adriana? Did you try any of this work for yourself?*

ADRIANA: *A little bit.*

CLINICIAN: *What do you remember doing?*

ADRIANA: *One day last week, I had to stay late for work, which means that I needed to call and ask my friend who lives in our apartment complex to pick up Lucas and Ana in front of the building where the school bus drops them off. After I got them from my friend's apartment and went to our place, I was frustrated and upset because I didn't like having to ask my friend to do that.*

CLINICIAN: *So, what negative thoughts did you have as part of your frustration?*

ADRIANA: *I remember thinking, "I hate my job." But then, I asked myself the positive opposite question. And guess what? I actually love my job.*

CLINICIAN: *How interesting.*

ADRIANA: *I know! So, when I kept saying that to myself, my mood got better, and I was also able to remember that my friend has no problems picking up the kids when I ask her to because she has to get her son, Jack, at the bus stop anyway. And Jack and Lucas are really good friends.*

CLINICIAN: *You also seem to be on the right track with learning how to identify and change your negative thoughts to positive ones.*

ADRIANA: *I think you're right. But, I have a lot of work to do before I get good at it.*

CLINICIAN: *Again, that's OK. The most important point is that both Lucas and you are making progress in learning how to do this. As always, the more you two practice, the better you'll both get. Also, remember that coming up with evidence or facts to support the positive thoughts is another part of the work.*

ADRIANA: *Thanks for the reminder.*

CLINICIAN: *You're welcome. So, before we finish for today, let's go over what we discussed. First, continue practicing with Lucas with either mild- or moderate-intensity emotions. Second, introduce the app as an additional regulating activity for him to learn how to use. Third, continue to work with Lucas to help him learn to identify and change his negative cognitions tied to his emotions, which can be aided by using the Emotion Identification Worksheet as a guide. Fourth, work on improving your own emotion regulation skills by continuing to identify and change your emotion-related cognitions. Any last questions before we end?*

ADRIANA: *Not really.*

CLINICIAN: *So, for next time, I want you to bring Lucas with you. I want to hear from him about all the work he's been doing the past several weeks, as well as all the progress he's been making. I also want to know if he has any questions for me that I can answer. Because school is such an important part of his life, I also want to hear from him and you, Adriana, how he's been doing in school lately and how well he's been regulating his emotions there. Finally, I want to talk to both of you about how the practicing and learning you've been doing is a specific example of what is called problem-solving. I want to describe to you both how a problem-solving approach can be used as a general life skill to help you get through challenging or difficult situations. Are you OK with bringing Lucas in with you next week?*

ADRIANA: *Definitely.*

CLINICIAN: *Perfect. See you next time. And remember, practice makes permanent.*

To review, here is what was covered in the session:

- The clinician verified that emotion regulation practice was conducted
- The clinician determined that the parent introduced a new regulating activity to their child
- The clinician ascertained that further practice with emotion regulation is warranted
- The clinician reviewed with the parent how they initially talked to their child about the cognitive component of emotions, including the introduction of the term, "self-talk"
- The clinician determined that the parent discussed with their child how changing negative cognitions to positive ones is another means to regulate emotions, which can be effected by the question, *"What's the positive opposite?"*
- The clinician described how the parent and their child can use the Emotion Identification Worksheet as a tool to help the child with continued practice to identify and change their negative cognitions
- The clinician reviewed how evidence can be gathered and used to support positive cognitions
- The clinician reminded the parent to reinforce their child for practicing and doing the work
- The clinician confirmed that the parent did some work to identify and change their own negative cognitions to regulate their emotions better
- The clinician emphasized continued practice to the parent in reappraising their own emotion-related cognitions
- The clinician requested that the parent bring their child to the next and last session for final discussions, including a problem-solving approach and closure

Session 7 - Emotion Regulation Training, Cognitive Restructuring, & Problem-Solving

> At the end of the session, the parent will be able to:
>
> - Facilitate and help maintain their child's newly acquired emotion regulation skills
> - Continue cognitive restructuring practice with their child and themselves
> - Troubleshoot future concerns by taking a problem-solving approach

This final session includes the parent and child. The child will have the opportunity to share their perspective on the work that they've been conducting to enhance their emotion regulation skills by engaging in a regulating activity and changing their emotion-related cognitions. The child and parent will also be requested to comment on the child's recent experiences in school and to what extent they've been able to regulate their emotions in that setting. The clinician will conclude the session by introducing and describing how the practice and work they've been conducting is an example of a problem-solving approach. The clinician will then explain how problem-solving, in general, can be used to address future concerns of the child, parent, or family. This discussion will be grounded in the seminal work conducted by Kazdin et al. (1992, 2003) in problem-solving skills training.

CLINICIAN: *Hi Lucas! It's great to see you and your mom today. I've heard from her that you've been working really hard to learn how to handle and cope with your emotions better. How do you think you've been doing?*

LUCAS: *Good. I think.*

ADRIANA: *Tell [Clinician's name] what you've been doing with the kinetic sand.*

LUCAS: *Oh yeah. I think the kinetic sand's awesome! I play with it as much as PLUS PLUS.*

CLINICIAN: *So, you've been using the sand to help make yourself feel better emotionally?*

LUCAS: *Uh-huh.*

CLINICIAN: *That is awesome, Lucas. Good for you. I'm really proud of you for practicing and learning how to use the blocks and sand as a way to cope with your negative emotions. Are you proud of yourself for learning how to do this?*

LUCAS: *Maybe.*

CLINICIAN: *Well, you should be. You're the one who's done the hard work and learned how to help yourself when your emotions are challenging. But, we should also remember that your mom has helped you with the practicing.*

ADRIANA: *Although that's right, you should be proud of yourself, Lucas, because you've been doing a great job.*

LUCAS: *Thanks, Mom.*

CLINICIAN: *Now, I'm wondering if you've tried using that relaxation app your mom downloaded onto her mobile phone.*

LUCAS: *A couple of times. I'm still trying to figure it out.*

CLINICIAN: *Tell me more, Lucas. What's it all about?*

LUCAS: *You're supposed to watch these videos they call "missions" that have animals in them.*

CLINICIAN: *Sounds interesting. My understanding is that the missions are different ways to relax and calm down. How much do you like the missions so far?*

LUCAS: *They're OK.*

CLINICIAN: *I'll take "OK," Lucas. Your mom probably told you that having a few activities to choose from to help yourself feel better emotionally is really important. Also, my guess is that if you keep practicing, you'll get so good at the missions that you won't have to watch the videos anymore to do them. Do you think I'm right?*

LUCAS: *I don't know.*

ADRIANA: *I think so, Lucas. Even after a couple of times, you're already starting to pick it up.*

CLINICIAN: *That's great to hear. My hope is that once you get good enough, you'll be able to use the missions in places besides your apartment, like school. That reminds me, how well have you been able to handle your emotions in school?*

LUCAS: *My teacher lets me take a break when I get mad with my schoolwork.*

ADRIANA: *That's because I talked to his teacher a couple of weeks ago and told him about the practicing Lucas has been doing with the blocks.*

CLINICIAN: *Good for you, Adriana! What do you do during your breaks, Lucas?*

LUCAS: *I go to the corner of our classroom where there's games and books and other stuff to do.*

CLINICIAN: *Is there PLUS PLUS or kinetic sand?*

LUCAS: *Nuh-uh. But, there's other kinds of blocks and things that I play with.*

CLINICIAN: *So, when you take a break, how much better do you feel emotionally?*

LUCAS: *A lot.*

CLINICIAN: *That's exactly what I was hoping for. Again, I'm very proud of you, Lucas. Now, I'm wondering about recess. I heard from your mom that sometimes you don't play with your classmates or friends and just sit to the side by yourself. Is that true?*

LUCAS: *Uh-huh.*

CLINICIAN: *What makes you do that?*

LUCAS: *I get sad when the other kids don't want to play with me.*

CLINICIAN: *So, your sadness can get in the way of having fun during recess. I know that your mom started working with you about self-talk or thoughts that go along with your emotions. Do you remember what you say to yourself when you're feeling sad during recess?*

LUCAS: *"The kids don't like me."*

CLINICIAN: *That makes total sense to me. Now, I'm going to ask you what I told your mom to do. What's the positive opposite of "The kids don't like me?"*

LUCAS: *"The kids like me."*

CLINICIAN: *Perfect, Lucas! Can you think of anything that shows the kids do like you?*

LUCAS: *They talk to me during lunch.*

CLINICIAN: *That's a great example of a fact or evidence that shows that they like you. Anything else you can think of?*

LUCAS: *Some of them are my friends.*

CLINICIAN: *If they don't really like you, they wouldn't be your friends, would they?*

LUCAS: *Uh-huh.*

CLINICIAN: *Well, it sounds like you're learning to identify the self-talk connected to your emotions and to change those negative thoughts to positive self-talk. Good for you, Lucas! If you keep practicing this, you will have another way to help yourself feel better emotionally.*
Let's talk about the relaxation app some more. When you experience sadness during recess, do you think that you can learn to use the missions in that situation to help make yourself feel better?

LUCAS: *I don't know.*

ADRIANA: *That's a great idea! In situations like that where there's nothing around to hold and do something with, you're going to need to do something by yourself, Lucas, without anything at all.*

CLINICIAN: *Exactly!*

LUCAS: *I guess I'll try then.*

CLINICIAN: *All I ask, Lucas, is for you to try your best. Because of how well you've practiced and learned so far, I'm confident that you will learn the missions and be able to use them in lots of situations. Like I've told you before, practice makes permanent, which means that you'll be able to do it for the rest of your life.*

ADRIANA: *I really think you can do it too, Lucas.*

CLINICIAN: *Great! Good luck then, Lucas, as you learn to use the missions.*
Before we end today's meeting, I want to talk to both of you about something else. It's called problem-solving. Actually, the practicing and work you've been doing is an example of a problem-solving approach. Whenever we experience a negative emotion, we are having some type of problem. The negative or bad feeling is simply telling us that something's not right. So, once we figure out that we have a problem, the first step in problem-solving is to ask ourselves the question, "What am I supposed to do?" Let's use an example. Lucas, when you get angry with your math homework, what are you supposed to do?

LUCAS: *Finish my homework.*

CLINICIAN: *That's right. Next, the second step is to say to ourselves, "I need to figure out what to do and what would happen." But, what if you can't continue doing your homework because your anger is getting too strong?*

LUCAS: *I can ask my mom to help me.*

ADRIANA: *You can always do that, Lucas, although sometimes I might not be able to help you right away because I'm busy with something else.*

CLINICIAN: *And that is related to the third step, which is asking the question, "Can I figure out what to do by myself?" If you think you can, then great. But, remember that you can always ask someone to help you if you think that you can't figure out what to do by yourself. Does that make sense, Lucas?*

LUCAS: *Uh-huh.*

CLINICIAN: *Like your mom said, sometimes she might not be able to help you right away. In the situation with your math homework, what one thing could you do and what would happen?*

LUCAS: *I could try to finish my homework. But I'd probably run to the stairs outside our apartment because I'd be too mad.*

CLINICIAN: *I can see that happening. So, what's another thing you could do and what would happen?*

LUCAS: *I could go to my room and play with the sand. Then, I wouldn't be so mad.*

CLINICIAN: *And that's exactly what you've been practicing, Lucas, and getting quite good at. Make sure that you come up with at least two things you could do before going to the next step. There's an old saying that's still true today—"There's usually more than one way to solve a problem." So, that leads us to the fourth step, which is to say to yourself, "I need to make a choice." Based on what you told your mom and me, what would you choose to do—continue with your homework or play with the sand?*

LUCAS: *Play with the sand.*

ADRIANA: *Which is what you've been doing the past couple of weeks when your math homework's been hard for you.*

CLINICIAN: *That's awesome, Lucas! You really have gotten good at helping yourself feel better emotionally. Now, to the fifth and final step—saying to yourself, "I need to find out how I did." Let's ask your mom about this one. Adriana, when Lucas ended up playing with the blocks or sand the past couple of weeks, did he go back and finish his math homework?*

ADRIANA: *Every single time. He's been amazing!*

LUCAS: *Thanks, Mom.*

ADRIANA: *I love you, Lucas.*

CLINICIAN: *So, that's it. Those are the five steps to problem-solving. Even though we used the example of an emotion-related problem, this approach can be used to work on any problem in our lives. And it doesn't matter if you're a kid, teenager, or an adult like you or me,*

Adriana. The way that I think about problem-solving is it gives us a set of instructions to figure things out when life gets hard, and we don't know exactly what to do. We can either solve problems on our own by following the steps or ask for help when we think that we need it. Just like before, you'll need to practice these steps to get good at problem-solving.

ADRIANA: *I think I'm going to practice this approach. As a single parent, things come up sometimes that I just don't know how to handle. But, these steps might make it easier for me to deal with and get less upset.*

CLINICIAN: *That's great to hear, Adriana! I'll give you an information sheet that lists all the steps* (see Appendix D). *I recommend that you practice problem-solving by using the sheet and doing so where Lucas can see and hear you. That way, you will be modeling how to do it, which is one of the main ways we learn—imitating what others do. In other words, you will be a role model for him as you become an effective problem solver.*

ADRIANA: *That's a wonderful idea!*

CLINICIAN: *At this point, I think that both of you have made lots of progress. Lucas, you've gotten pretty good at helping yourself feel better emotionally when you're experiencing negative emotions like anger, sadness, and worry or anxiety. And Adriana, you've gotten really good at helping Lucas better regulate his emotions. So, because I'm quite confident that both of you know what to do and how to practice, I don't think that we need to continue to meet right now. But, if things come up in the future and you feel that you want my help, please feel free to reach out to me, and we can schedule a follow-up session. How does that sound to you two?*

ADRIANA: *Sounds good to me.*

LUCAS: *Me too.*

CLINICIAN: *So, goodbye for now. I have been honored to work with you both.*

To review, here is what was covered in the session:

- The clinician assessed from the child's perspective how they've been doing with the practicing to enhance their emotion regulation skills by engaging in regulating activities
- The clinician informed the child and parent that possessing and utilizing several regulating activities are beneficial
- The clinician assessed from the child's perspective how well they've been doing in school, especially in regard to regulating their emotions
- From the child's perspective, the clinician assessed how much they'd learned thus far in identifying and changing their emotion-related cognitions

- The clinician introduced problem solving and described how practicing and engaging in emotion regulation are aligned with a problem-solving approach
- The clinician reviewed each step of problem-solving
- The clinician recommended to the parent to practice problem-solving in the child's presence to be a role model for them in learning the strategy
- The clinician, parent, and child collaboratively terminated treatment (for the time being)

6

Final Thoughts .... and Skills

At the end of this chapter, you will be able to:

- Train parents how to generalize their children's emotion regulation skills
  - Across stimuli
  - Across emotions and related behaviors
  - Across social settings
  - Across physical environments
- Collaborate with the parent and child to identify developmentally appropriate activities for use in emotion regulation
- Help parents to learn how to identify and manage risk
  - Intrapersonal and interpersonal factors
  - Familial processes
  - External and systems issues: peers, school, neighborhood, and community

Parenting from a Lifelong Learning Perspective

As of this writing, the world has endured almost two years of the COVID-19 pandemic. This global adversity has impacted the lives of millions of children and their families, and time (and research) will tell what the long-term health consequences are. As we learned from the earlier chapters of this book, exposure to developmental adversity sets the stage for developing significant behavioral health problems. In a national survey of parents in the United States a couple of months after the onset of the pandemic, 27% reported worsening behavioral health for themselves, and 14% reported declining behavioral health for their children (Patrick et al., 2020). In the context of this mass or collective adversity, supporting and nurturing our children's behavioral health are perhaps as urgent and needed as ever.

Trauma-Informed Parenting Program: TIP^s for Clinicians to Train Parents of Children Impacted by Trauma & Adversity, First Edition. Carryl P. Navalta.
© 2022 John Wiley & Sons, Inc. Published 2022 by John Wiley & Sons, Inc.
Companion Website: www.wiley.com/go/navalta/tipsforclinicians

The cornerstone of this book is that parents have the capacity to help their children regulate their emotions and related behaviors. For children who experience emotion dysregulation secondary to exposure to adverse childhood experiences (ACEs), this role is vital to their development. The ACE Study and others have elucidated a developmental pathway in which a child who has experienced significant adversity will lead a challenging life, later peppered with chronic health problems and social problems. Unfortunately, this path can also be a deadly one because the odds are that this person will die prematurely in adulthood. Through a prevention lens, we need to get such children off this path as early as possible to avoid adverse outcomes regardless of where they are along the path. Improving children's ability to regulate emotions and related behaviors is one way to potentially alter their life trajectories. Again, parents can serve as a prominent function in this process.

Clinicians working with parents may need to provide further therapeutic services above and beyond the treatment detailed in this manual. For one, the foundational skills may not be fully actualized when the initial treatment is conducted. Second, regression may occur, thus requiring follow-up booster sessions to re-establish the child's previously acquired skills. Third, the child's emotion regulation skills may not generalize across one or more aspects. Although the treatment described herein focused on the home setting, directly involving the child's teacher was also highlighted. However, clinical experience and research have demonstrated that the generalization of newly acquired skills must be planned for and not assumed.

Generalization of Skills

The guiding principle of generalization is the notion of sufficient exemplars. A minimum number of examples of a particular feature of a given skill must be practiced and learned so that a pattern emerges and becomes instilled in the individual. Although this minimum is typically not predictable beforehand, the number usually decreases as the child's developmental maturity increases. Several features exist in which sufficient exemplars must be learned for generalization to occur. One of these features is the stimulus that elicits the specific emotion. As a reminder, a stimulus emanates from a source of stimulation. For example, the elicitation of emotions can be stimulated by sources of threat, antagonism, loss, wrongdoing, and the like. The second characteristic is the actual emotion(s) and related behavior(s). When aligned with the sources of stimulation just outlined, the core emotions include anxiety, anger, sadness, and guilt or shame, respectively. Third, generalization of skills typically cannot occur unless the practicing and learning are conducted in multiple social settings. Specifically, the skill needs to be exhibited in the presence of various people to the point that their presence no longer matters, and the child can use the skill independent of the individuals around them. Lastly, the skill requires practice in multiple physical environments as well.

Although such learning may indirectly occur when varied social settings are targeted for generalization, exemplars of physical surroundings must also be established. Ultimately, the clinician is the one who is responsible for determining to what extent the child's emotion regulation skills have generalized. If generalization is insufficient, the clinician must decide how to best intervene by incorporating enough examples of the characteristics described above. When successful, the child will possess a skill set that is both effective and robust.

Developmentally Appropriate Therapeutic Activities

As outlined in Chapter 5, the treatment highlighted parent training focused on a child at a certain age (nine years) and within a specific developmental window (middle childhood). Thus, the activities identified and utilized for emotion regulation were appropriate to the child's level of development. For children who are younger or older, the issue then is what activities the clinician should consider when deciding what the parent should be practicing with their child. Children have varied interests in what captures their attention and gratifies them. These activities also typically match children's cognitive and socioemotional development. They also need to be acceptable to parents and other caregiving or supportive adults in the child's life. Although the number of possible activities can be initially daunting, the clinician is guided by certain key qualities. As a reminder, these properties include the following:

- Elicits internal positivity
- Done independently
- Conducted for several minutes, uninterrupted
- Performed relatively quietly
- Carried out in a sedentary/seated position

Although screen-based games (e.g., computer, video, mobile phone) can meet these requirements, they typically should be avoided, given that excitability is often elicited. Such a state could perpetuate or even potentiate the physiological arousal component of negative emotions, especially when their intensity levels are relatively high. Instead, regulating activities should dampen the emotion-related arousal. As long as the clinician collaborates with the parent and child, they should be able to identify a few developmentally appropriate activities that the child can learn to use to regulate their negative emotions. Once the parent recognizes the types of activities that can be regulating for the child, they will be positioned well to continue facilitating their child's identification of new regulating activities as the child develops and matures. Perhaps even more importantly, the child will eventually develop the capacity to identify future activities to be used for regulation independently. In many ways, this process can be understood as a form of self-care: *"the ability of individuals, families, and communities to promote health, prevent disease, maintain health, and to **cope with illness and disability** with or without the support of a healthcare provider"* (emphasis added; World Health Organization, 2009).

One issue that sometimes comes up with parents is that allowing their children to engage in regulating activities essentially permits them to avoid or escape their responsibilities. At the outset, this perspective is reasonable, especially in situations where the child ends up not participating in an activity or event in which their engagement at the moment is expected, such as schoolwork. Some parents thus worry that the child will learn to "act out" as a means to get out of or escape from a non- or less-preferred activity. In other words, their expressed emotion dysregulation is predicted to evolve to escape-motivated behavior.

However, this tenet doesn't take into consideration two integral points. First, emotion dysregulation in children exposed to developmental adversity is a deficiency or deficit in a core regulatory process due to disrupted development. Therefore, engaging in an activity that elicits internal positivity is, in effect, activating this regulatory process enhanced by practice and learning through parent training. Second, "escape" from any current situation is a temporary one because the child transitions to a more regulated state that allows them to return to the activity or event at hand. If the child is not allowed to regulate their emotions, they would not be engaged in the activity anyway because their capacity to do so would be compromised by the negative emotions experienced at the time. Although the premise that the child can learn to "act out" to escape from a current situation and engage in a more-preferred activity is improbable, the clinician will need to monitor and assess this possibility as the parent training is conducted.

Protect and Help: Two Vital Roles of Parents

Returning to the concept of the trauma system, two critical functions bear mentioning: protection and help. One of the most fundamental roles of parents (i.e., family system) of children impacted by ACEs is protecting them from perceived threat and danger sources and significant life stressors. Because the children are especially sensitive to negative emotional stimuli, preventing them from being cued by such stimulation minimizes their risk of experiencing dysregulated emotions and related behavior. Through the parent training described in this book, parents can learn about the types of stimuli that can elicit their child's dysregulation. With this knowledge, they can then learn with the clinician's assistance to anticipate when sources of such stimulation may become manifest and thus prevent their child's exposure to them. However, preventing children's exposure to all stimuli is an impossibility. Therefore, when such exposure is unpreventable or unavoidable, the help function of the trauma system needs to come into play. This function is fundamentally what this book is all about—teaching parents to help their children navigate the terrain when life brings about hurdles and obstacles leading to wants and needs not being met.

By extension, parents need to activate the protection and help functions for their entire family unit (themselves included) when required. As we've learned in this book, emotional stimuli can emanate from varied sources of stimulation. For each individual, what elicits their emotions can be unique to them, thus distinct from others. Another role of the clinician then is to work with parents to help them learn where sources of perceived threat and danger and life stress may lie. Here, the clinician has another set of guidelines introduced in this book to follow—namely, the proximal-to-distal layers of social ecologies in which we inhabit.

Intrapersonal or intrinsic factors need to be identified and acknowledged at the closest layer. Such processes are best exemplified by the presence of acute or chronic health problems that can serve as significant stressors for parents. Clinicians need to advocate for parents who have health problems that limit or interfere with their ability to support and nurture their children if they are not receiving the proper care they need to treat the problems, regardless of whether the problems are physical or behavioral. Another approach is for the clinician to teach the parent how to advocate for themselves to access healthcare.

The next layer is a related one in which the parents' ability to socialize and interact with others is less than adequate relative to same-age peers. This compromised capacity can then lead to interpersonal problems as another source of stress. In this case, the clinician needs to decide how the parent's interpersonal effectiveness can be enhanced, such as directly working with the parent to improve social skills. Within the family unit (the next layer of the social ecology), sources of stress or emotional stimuli can also exist. If the clinician determines that family members beyond the targeted child (or even the whole family) are essentially not functioning adequately, then a systems approach to working with the family may be warranted (Champine et al., 2018).

Lastly, sources of stress can be present across several layers external to the family, including peers, school, neighborhood, and community. Again, the clinician needs to work with the parent to help them learn how to identify such sources and advocate for themselves and their family to address the issues. Problems within the school system illustrate how sources of stress can exist. Because success in this life domain is vital to children's development, working with the parents from an advocacy approach is again required, such as informing them about children's rights to a free and appropriate education regardless of disability status. Once parents understand where risks can arise, they will be better positioned to protect and help their loved ones and themselves.

Conclusion: Being Healthy to Living Fully

The overarching purpose of this book is to support and facilitate children's development of emotion regulation by capitalizing on parents' influence on their children's regulatory processes. The ability to regulate emotions and related behavior is a foundational life skill that promotes health and wellness, both short- and long-term. In the context of the COVID-19 pandemic, much time, effort, and money have been spent keeping people worldwide healthy and preventing them from becoming ill from the disease. Thus, good or optimal health has been labeled as the goal in almost all discussions. However, one individual, Dr. Sandro Galea, Dean of the School of Public Health at Boston University, has illuminated an alternative goal that arguably needs to be front and center. Rather than being healthy as a state to achieve and maintain over time as the ultimate outcome, living a fulfilling life should be what counts most. As Dr. Galea (2021) eloquently stated:

> *"Health matters because love matters, because connection matters, because working with valued colleagues matters, because tasting food matters, because going for a swim matters, because traveling abroad matters, because watching your daughter graduate from college matters, because writing a book matters, because living a rich, full life matters—which we cannot do unless we are healthy."*

With a little bit of luck and a lot of hard work, children exposed to developmental adversity can live their lives in the ways that matter to them. Hopefully, this book will help such children along the way.

Appendix A

Case Conceptualization Development Form

Primary Problem Template

When (child's name) is triggered by (source of stimulation and emotional stimuli perceived), they/she/he react by engaging in (emotion-related behaviors). As a result, (child's name) experiences (activity limitations and participation restrictions). These constraints have put them/her/him at risk for (psychosocial or functional impairment [or physical harm when appropriate]).

3 Ps	Assessment Modality	Treatment-Related Factors	Assessment Modality
Predisposing Factors 1._____ 2._____ 3._____ 4._____	□ Clinical interview □ Rating scales □ Direct observation □ Self-monitoring □ Clinical records review □ Other: _____	Personal Strengths 1._____ 2._____ 3._____ 4._____	□ Clinical interview □ Rating scales □ Direct observation □ Self-monitoring □ Clinical records review □ Other: _____
Precipitating Factors 1._____ 2._____ 3._____ 4._____	□ Clinical interview □ Rating scales □ Direct observation □ Self-monitoring □ Clinical records review □ Other: _____	External Resources/Assets 1._____ 2._____ 3._____ 4._____	□ Clinical interview □ Rating scales □ Direct observation □ Self-monitoring □ Clinical records review □ Other: _____
Perpetuating Factors 1._____ 2._____ 3._____ 4._____	□ Clinical interview □ Rating scales □ Direct observation □ Self-monitoring □ Clinical records review □ Other: _____	Problems 1._____ 2._____ 3._____ 4._____	□ Clinical interview □ Rating scales □ Direct observation □ Self-monitoring □ Clinical records review □ Other: _____

Trauma-Informed Parenting Program: TIP^s for Clinicians to Train Parents of Children Impacted by Trauma & Adversity, First Edition. Carryl P. Navalta.
© 2022 John Wiley & Sons, Inc. Published 2022 by John Wiley & Sons, Inc.
Companion Website: www.wiley.com/go/navalta/tipsforclinicians

Appendix B

Treatment Planning Form

Long-Term Goal Template

At the end of treatment, when (child's name) is triggered by (source of stimulation and emotional stimuli perceived), they/she/he react by engaging less in (emotion-related behaviors). As a result, (child's name) experiences greater participation in (activities, events, or situations). This increased engagement puts them/her/him at higher chances for (psychosocial or functional improvement).

Goals (one for each primary problem)

1. _____
   _____
   _____
   _____

2. _____
   _____
   _____
   _____

3. _____
   _____
   _____
   _____

4. _____
   _____
   _____
   _____

Trauma-Informed Parenting Program: TIP⁵ for Clinicians to Train Parents of Children Impacted by Trauma & Adversity, First Edition. Carryl P. Navalta.
© 2022 John Wiley & Sons, Inc. Published 2022 by John Wiley & Sons, Inc.
Companion Website: www.wiley.com/go/navalta/tipsforclinicians

Short-Term Objective Template

After (# weeks/months) of treatment, when (child's name) is triggered by (source of stimulation and emotional stimuli perceived), they/she/he react by engaging less (frequency, duration, and/or intensity) in (emotion-related behaviors). As a result, (child's name) experiences greater participation (frequency, duration) in (activities, events, or situations).

Objectives (one for each goal)

1. _____
_____
_____

2. _____
_____
_____

3. _____
_____
_____

4. _____
_____
_____

Interventions (at least one for each objective)

1. _____
_____

2. _____
_____

3. _____
_____

4. _____
_____

Diagnosis (DSM or ICD)

1. _____

2. _____

3. _____

4. _____

Appendix C

Emotion Identification Worksheet

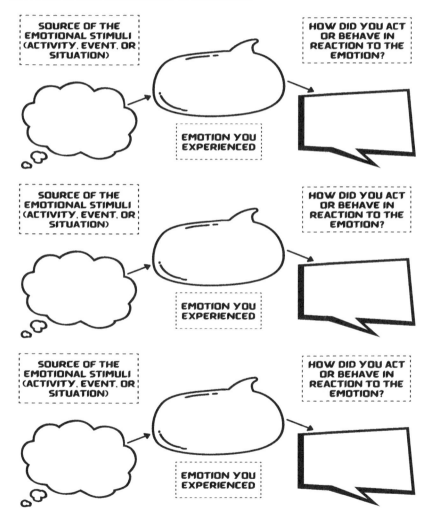

Trauma-Informed Parenting Program: TIP^s for Clinicians to Train Parents of Children Impacted by Trauma & Adversity, First Edition. Carryl P. Navalta.
© 2022 John Wiley & Sons, Inc. Published 2022 by John Wiley & Sons, Inc.
Companion Website: www.wiley.com/go/navalta/tipsforclinicians

Appendix D

Problem-Solving Steps

1) "What am I supposed to do?"
2) "Can I figure out what to do by myself?"
3) "I need to figure out what to do and what would happen."
4) "I need to make a choice."
5) "I need to find out how I did."

Adapted from: Kazdin, A. E. (2017). Parent management training and problem-solving skills training for child and adolescent conduct problems. In J. R. Weisz & A. E. Kazdin (Eds.). *Evidence-based psychotherapies for children and adolescents* (3rd ed., pp. 142–158). Guilford Press.

Trauma-Informed Parenting Program: TIP^s for Clinicians to Train Parents of Children Impacted by Trauma & Adversity, First Edition. Carryl P. Navalta.
© 2022 John Wiley & Sons, Inc. Published 2022 by John Wiley & Sons, Inc.
Companion Website: www.wiley.com/go/navalta/tipsforclinicians

References

Achenbach, T. M., McConaughy, S. H., & Howell, C. T. (1987). Child/adolescent behavioral and emotional problems: Implications of cross-informant correlations for situational specificity. *Psychological Bulletin, 101*(2), 213–232. https://doi.org/10.1037/0033-2909.101.2.213

Alisic, E., Conroy, R., & Thoresen, S. (2020). Epidemiology, clinical presentation, and developmental considerations in children and adolescents. In D. Forbes, J. I. Bisson, C. M. Monson, & L. Berliner (Eds.), *Effective treatments for PTSD: Practice guidelines from the International Society for Traumatic Stress Studies* (3rd ed., pp. 30–48). Guilford Publications.

Alisic, E., Zalta, A. K., van Wesel, F., Larsen, S. E., Hafstad, G. S., Hassanpour, K., & Smid, G. E. (2014). Rates of post-traumatic stress disorder in trauma-exposed children and adolescents: Meta-analysis. *British Journal of Psychiatry, 204*(5), 335–340. https://doi.org/10.1192/bjp.bp.113.131227

American Psychiatric Association. (2000). *Diagnostic and statistical manual of mental disorders: DSM-IV-TR* (4th ed., text rev.).

American Psychiatric Association. (2013a). *Diagnostic and statistical manual of mental disorders: DSM-5* (5th ed.). https://doi.org/10.1176/appi.books .9780890425596

American Psychiatric Association. (2013b). *Cultural formulation interview.* file:/// Users/cnavalta/Downloads/APA_DSM5_Cultural-Formulation-Interview.pdf

Andersen, S. L. (2015). Exposure to early adversity: Points of cross-species translation that can lead to improved understanding of depression. *Development and Psychopathology, 27*(2), 477–491. https://doi.org/10.1017/ S0954579415000103

Askevold, F. (1976). War sailor syndrome. *Psychotherapy and Psychosomatics, 27*(3–6), 133–138. https://doi.org/10.1159/000287009

Ayoub, C. C., O'Connor, E., Rappolt-Schlichtmann, G., Fischer, K. W., Rogosch, F. A., Toth, S. L., & Cicchetti, D. (2006). Cognitive and emotional differences in young maltreated children: A translational application of dynamic skill theory. *Development and Psychopathology, 18*(03). https://doi.org/10.1017/ S0954579406060342

Bailey, B. N., Delaney-Black, V., Hannigan, J. H., Ager, J., Sokol, R. J., & Covington, C. Y. (2005). Somatic complaints in children and community violence exposure. *Journal of Developmental and Behavioral Pediatrics: JDBP, 26*(5), 341–348. https://doi.org/10.1097/00004703-200510000-00001

Barron, I. G., Bourgaize, C., Lempertz, D., Swinden, C., & Darker-Smith, S. (2019). Eye movement desensitization reprocessing for children and adolescents with posttraumatic stress disorder: A systematic narrative review. *Journal of EMDR Practice and Research, 13*(4), 270–283. https://doi.org/10.1891/1933-3196.13.4.270

Beauchaine, T. P. (2015). Future directions in emotion dysregulation and youth psychopathology. *Journal of Clinical Child & Adolescent Psychology, 44*(5), 875–896. https://doi.org/10.1080/15374416.2015.1038827

Belsky, J. (1993). Etiology of child maltreatment: A developmental-ecological analysis. *Psychological Bulletin, 114*(3), 413–434. https://doi.org/10.1037/0033-2909.114.3.413

Benner, A. D., Wang, Y., Shen, Y., Boyle, A. E., Polk, R., & Cheng, Y.-P. (2018). Racial/ethnic discrimination and well-being during adolescence: A meta-analytic review. *The American Psychologist, 73*(7), 855–883. https://doi.org/10.1037/amp0000204

Berliner, L., Meiser-Stedman, R., & Danese, A. (2020). Screening, assessment, and diagnosis in children and adolescents. In D. Forbes, J. I. Bisson, C. M. Monson, & L. Berliner (Eds.), *Effective treatments for PTSD: Practice guidelines from the International Society for Traumatic Stress Studies* (3rd ed., pp. 69–89). The Guilford Press.

Bethell, C. D., Newacheck, P., Hawes, E., & Halfon, N. (2014). Adverse childhood experiences: Assessing the impact on health and school engagement and the mitigating role of resilience. *Health Affairs, 33*(12), 2106–2115. https://doi.org/10.1377/hlthaff.2014.0914

Blaustein, M. E., & Kinniburgh, K. M. (2010). *Treating traumatic stress in children and adolescents: How to foster resilience through attachment, self-regulation, and competency.* Guilford Press.

Borrell-Carrió, F., Suchman, A. L., & Epstein, R. M. (2004). The biopsychosocial model 25 years later: Principles, practice, and scientific inquiry. *Annals of Family Medicine, 2*(6), 576–582. https://doi.org/10.1370/afm.245

Bosquet Enlow, M., Kassam-Adams, N., & Saxe, G. (2010). The child stress disorders checklist-short form: A four-item scale of traumatic stress symptoms in children. *General Hospital Psychiatry, 32*(3), 321–327. https://doi.org/10.1016/j.genhosppsych.2010.01.009

Briere, J. (1996). *Trauma symptom checklist for children (TSCC) professional manual.* Psychological Assessment Resources.

Briere, J., Johnson, K., Bissada, A., Damon, L., Crouch, J., Gil, E., Hanson, R., & Ernst, V. (2001). The trauma symptom checklist for young children (TSCYC): Reliability and association with abuse exposure in a multi-site study. *Child*

Abuse & Neglect, 25(8), 1001–1014. https://doi.org/10.1016/S0145-2134(01)00253-8

Briggs, E. C., Nooner, K., & Amaya-Jackson, L. (2014). Assessment of childhood PTSD. In M. J. Friedman, T. M. Keane, & P. A. Resick (Eds.), *Handbook of PTSD: Science and practice* (2nd ed., pp. 391–405). The Guilford Press.

Bronfenbrenner, U. (1977). Toward an experimental ecology of human development. *American Psychologist*, 32(7), 513–531. https://doi.org/10.1037/0003-066X.32.7.513

Bronfenbrenner, U. (1979). *The ecology of human development: Experiments by nature and design.* Harvard University Press.

Bronfenbrenner, U. (1995). Developmental ecology through space and time: A future perspective. In P. Moen, G. H. Elder, & K. Lüscher (Eds.), *Examining lives in context: Perspectives on the ecology of human development* (pp. 619–647). American Psychological Association. https://doi.org/10.1037/10176-018

Brown, A., Navalta, C. P., Tullberg, E., & Saxe, G. (2014). Trauma systems therapy: An approach to creating trauma-informed child welfare systems. In R. M. Reece, R. F. Hanson, & J. Sargent (Eds.), *Treatment of child abuse: Common ground for mental health, medical, and legal practitioners* (2nd ed., pp. 132–138). Johns Hopkins University Press.

Brown, E. J., Cohen, J. A., & Mannarino, A. P. (2020). Trauma-focused cognitive-behavioral therapy: The role of caregivers. *Journal of Affective Disorders*, 277, 39–45. https://doi.org/10.1016/j.jad.2020.07.123

Brown, J., Cohen, P., Johnson, J. G., & Smailes, E. M. (1999). Childhood abuse and neglect: Specificity of effects on adolescent and young adult depression and suicidality. *Journal of the American Academy of Child & Adolescent Psychiatry*, 38(12), 1490–1496. https://doi.org/10.1097/00004583-199912000-00009

Bulik, C. M., Prescott, C. A., & Kendler, K. S. (2001). Features of childhood sexual abuse and the development of psychiatric and substance use disorders. *British Journal of Psychiatry*, 179(5), 444–449. https://doi.org/10.1192/bjp.179.5.444

Burgess, A. W., & Holmstrom, L. L. (1974). Rape trauma syndrome. *American Journal of Psychiatry*, 131(9), 981–986. https://doi.org/10.1176/ajp.131.9.981

Call, N. A., Scheithauer, M. C., & Mevers, J. L. (2017). Functional behavioral assessments. In J. K. Luiselli (Ed.), *Applied behavior analysis advanced guidebook* (pp. 41–71). Elsevier. https://doi.org/10.1016/B978-0-12-811122-2.00003-6

Caspi, A., Sugden, K., Moffitt, T. E., Taylor, A., Craig, I. W., Harrington, H., McClay, J., Mill, J., Martin, J., Braithwaite, A., & Poulton, R. (2003). Influence of life stress on depression: Moderation by a polymorphism in the 5-HTT Gene. *Science*, 301(5631), 386–389. https://doi.org/10.1126/science.1083968

Center on the Developing Child. (n.d.). *How racism can affect child development*. Harvard University. https://developingchild.harvard.edu/resources/racism-and-ecd

Chaffin, M., & Shultz, S. K. (2001). Psychometric evaluation of the children's impact of traumatic events scale-revised. *Child Abuse & Neglect, 25*(3), 401–411. https://doi.org/10.1016/S0145-2134(00)00257-X

Champine, R. B., Matlin, S., Strambler, M. J., & Tebes, J. K. (2018). Trauma-informed family practices: Toward integrated and evidence-based approaches. *Journal of Child and Family Studies, 27*(9), 2732–2743. https://doi.org/10.1007/s10826-018-1118-0

Choi, J., Jeong, B., Rohan, M. L., Polcari, A. M., & Teicher, M. H. (2009). Preliminary evidence for white matter tract abnormalities in young adults exposed to parental verbal abuse. *Biological Psychiatry, 65*(3), 227–234. https://doi.org/10.1016/j.biopsych.2008.06.022

Choi, K. R., McCreary, M., Ford, J. D., Rahmanian Koushkaki, S., Kenan, K. N., & Zima, B. T. (2019). Validation of the traumatic events screening inventory for ACEs. *Pediatrics, 143*(4), e20182546. https://doi.org/10.1542/peds.2018-2546

Chorpita, B. F., Daleiden, E. L., Ebesutani, C., Young, J., Becker, K. D., Nakamura, B. J., Phillips, L., Ward, A., Lynch, R., Trent, L., Smith, R. L., Okamura, K., & Starace, N. (2011). Evidence-based treatments for children and adolescents: An updated review of indicators of efficacy and effectiveness. *Clinical Psychology: Science and Practice, 18*(2), 154–172. https://doi.org/10.1111/j.1468-2850.2011.01247.x

Chu, B. C. (2012). Translating transdiagnostic approaches to children and adolescents. *Cognitive and Behavioral Practice, 19*(1), 1–4. https://doi.org/10.1016/j.cbpra.2011.06.003

Cicchetti, D., & Handley, E. D. (2019). Child maltreatment and the development of substance use and disorder. *Neurobiology of Stress, 10*, 100144. https://doi.org/10.1016/j.ynstr.2018.100144

Cicchetti, D., & Lynch, M. (1993). Toward an ecological/transactional model of community violence and child maltreatment: Consequences for children's development. *Psychiatry, 56*(1), 96–118. https://doi.org/10.1080/00332747.1993.11024624

Cicchetti, D., & Valentino, K. (2015). An ecological-transactional perspective on child maltreatment: Failure of the average expectable environment and its influence on child development. In D. Cicchetti & D. J. Cohen (Eds.), *Developmental psychopathology* (pp. 129–201). John Wiley & Sons, Inc. https://doi.org/10.1002/9780470939406.ch4

Clark, R., Anderson, N. B., Clark, V. R., & Williams, D. R. (1999). Racism as a stressor for African Americans: A biopsychosocial model. *American Psychologist, 54*(10), 805–816. https://doi.org/10.1037/0003-066X.54.10.805

Coates, J., Taylor, J. A., & Sayal, K. (2015). Parenting interventions for ADHD: A systematic literature review and meta-analysis. *Journal of Attention Disorders, 19*(10), 831–843. https://doi.org/10.1177/1087054714535952

Cohen, J. A., Bukstein, O., Walter, H., Benson, S. R., Chrisman, A., Farchione, T. R., Hamilton, J., Keable, H., Kinlan, J., Schoettle, U., Siegel, M., Stock, S., & Medicus, J. & AACAP Work Group On Quality Issues (2010). Practice parameter for the assessment and treatment of children and adolescents with posttraumatic stress disorder. *Journal of the American Academy of Child and Adolescent Psychiatry, 49*(4), 414–430. https://doi.org/10.1016/j.jaac.2009.12.020

Cohen, L. R., Hien, D. A., & Batchelder, S. (2008). The impact of cumulative maternal trauma and diagnosis on parenting behavior. *Child Maltreatment, 13*(1), 27–38. https://doi.org/10.1177/1077559507310045

Cole, P. M., Hall, S. E., & Hajal, N. (2017). Emotion dysregulation as a vulnerability to psychopathology. In T. P. Beauchaine & S. P. Hinshaw (Eds.), *Child and adolescent psychopathology* (3rd ed., pp. 346–386). John Wiley & Sons.

Collins, K. S., Strieder, F. H., DePanfilis, D., Tabor, M., Freeman, P. A. C., Linde, L., & Greenberg, P. (2011). Trauma adapted family connections: Reducing developmental and complex trauma symptomatology to prevent child abuse and neglect. *Child Welfare, 90*(6), 29–47. https://www.researchgate.net/publication/224845518_Trauma_Adapted_Family_Connections_Reducing_Developmental_and_Complex_Trauma_Symptomatology_to_Prevent_Child_Abuse_and_Neglect.

Compas, B. E., Jaser, S. S., Bettis, A. H., Watson, K. H., Gruhn, M. A., Dunbar, J. P., Williams, E., & Thigpen, J. C. (2017). Coping, emotion regulation, and psychopathology in childhood and adolescence: A meta-analysis and narrative review. *Psychological Bulletin, 143*(9), 939–991. https://doi.org/10.1037/bul0000110

Copeland, W. E., Keeler, G., Angold, A., & Costello, E. J. (2007). Traumatic events and posttraumatic stress in childhood. *Archives of General Psychiatry, 64*(5), 577. https://doi.org/10.1001/archpsyc.64.5.577

Cornelius, M. D., De Genna, N. M., Goldschmidt, L., Larkby, C., & Day, N. L. (2016). Prenatal alcohol and other early childhood adverse exposures: Direct and indirect pathways to adolescent drinking. *Neurotoxicology and Teratology, 55*, 8–15. https://doi.org/10.1016/j.ntt.2016.03.001

Cowell, R. A., Cicchetti, D., Rogosch, F. A., & Toth, S. L. (2015). Childhood maltreatment and its effect on neurocognitive functioning: Timing and chronicity matter. *Development and Psychopathology, 27*(2), 521–533. https://doi.org/10.1017/S0954579415000139

Cronholm, P. F., Forke, C. M., Wade, R., Bair-Merritt, M. H., Davis, M., Harkins-Schwarz, M., Pachter, L. M., & Fein, J. A. (2015). Adverse childhood experiences. *American Journal of Preventive Medicine, 49*(3), 354–361. https://doi.org/10.1016/j.amepre.2015.02.001

Crozier, J. C., & Barth, R. P. (2005). Cognitive and academic functioning in maltreated children. *Children & Schools, 27*(4), 197–206. https://doi.org/10.1093/cs/27.4.197

D'Andrea, W., Ford, J., Stolbach, B., Spinazzola, J., & van der Kolk, B. A. (2012). Understanding interpersonal trauma in children: Why we need a developmentally appropriate trauma diagnosis. *The American Journal of Orthopsychiatry, 82*(2), 187–200. https://doi.org/10.1111/j.1939-0025.2012.01154.x

Dalgleish, T., Meiser-Stedman, R., & Smith, P. (2005). Cognitive aspects of posttraumatic stress reactions and their treatment in children and adolescents: An empirical review and some recommendations. *Behavioural and Cognitive Psychotherapy, 33*(4), 459–486. https://doi.org/10.1017/S1352465805002389

de Figueiredo, C. S., Sandre, P. C., Portugal, L. C. L., Mázala-de-Oliveira, T., da Silva Chagas, L., Raony, Í., Ferreira, E. S., Giestal-de-Araujo, E., Dos Santos, A. A., & Bomfim, P. O.-S. (2021). COVID-19 pandemic impact on children and adolescents' mental health: Biological, environmental, and social factors. *Progress in Neuro-Psychopharmacology & Biological Psychiatry, 106*, 110171. https://doi.org/10.1016/j.pnpbp.2020.110171

De Los Reyes, A., Augenstein, T. M., & Aldao, A. (2018). Assessment issues in child and adolescent psychotherapy. In J. R. Weisz & A. E. Kazdin (Eds.), *Evidence-based psychotherapies for children and adolescents* (3rd ed., pp. 537–554). The Guilford Press.

De Los Reyes, A., Augenstein, T. M., Wang, M., Thomas, S. A., Drabick, D. A. G., Burgers, D. E., & Rabinowitz, J. (2015). The validity of the multi-informant approach to assessing child and adolescent mental health. *Psychological Bulletin, 141*(4), 858–900. https://doi.org/10.1037/a0038498

de Paúl, J., & Arruabarrena, M. I. (1995). Behavior problems in school-aged physically abused and neglected children in Spain. *Child Abuse & Neglect, 19*(4), 409–418. https://doi.org/10.1016/0145-2134(95)00009-W

DePierro, J., D'Andrea, W., Spinazzola, J., Stafford, E., van Der Kolk, B., Saxe, G., Stolbach, B., McKernan, S., & Ford, J. D. (2019). Beyond PTSD: Client presentations of developmental trauma disorder from a national survey of clinicians. *Psychological Trauma: Theory, Research, Practice and Policy.* https://doi.org/10.1037/tra0000532

Dirkzwager, A. J. E., Kerssens, J. J., & Yzermans, C. J. (2006). Health problems in children and adolescents before and after a man-made disaster. *Journal of the American Academy of Child & Adolescent Psychiatry, 45*(1), 94–103. https://doi.org/10.1097/01.chi.0000186402.05465.f7

Djeddah, C., Facchin, P., Ranzato, C., & Romer, C. (2000). Child abuse: Current problems and key public health challenges. *Social Science & Medicine, 51*(6), 905–915. https://doi.org/10.1016/S0277-9536(00)00070-8

Dorn, T., Yzermans, J. C., Spreeuwenberg, P. M. M., Schilder, A., & van der Zee, J. (2008). A cohort study of the long-term impact of a fire disaster on the physical and mental health of adolescents. *Journal of Traumatic Stress, 21*(2), 239–242. https://doi.org/10.1002/jts.20328

Dorsey, S., McLaughlin, K. A., Kerns, S. E. U., Harrison, J. P., Lambert, H. K., Briggs, E. C., Revillion Cox, J., & Amaya-Jackson, L. (2017). Evidence base update for psychosocial treatments for children and adolescents exposed to traumatic events. *Journal of Clinical Child and Adolescent Psychology: The Official Journal for the Society of Clinical Child and Adolescent Psychology, American Psychological Association, Division 53, 46*(3), 303–330. https://doi.org/10.1080/15374416.2016.1220309

Dvir, Y., Ford, J. D., Hill, M., & Frazier, J. A. (2014). Childhood maltreatment, emotional dysregulation, and psychiatric comorbidities. *Harvard Review of Psychiatry, 22*(3), 149–161. https://doi.org/10.1097/HRP.0000000000000014

Eckenrode, J., Laird, M., & Doris, J. (1993). School performance and disciplinary problems among abused and neglected children. *Developmental Psychology, 29*(1), 53–62. https://doi.org/10.1037/0012-1649.29.1.53

Eckshtain, D., Kuppens, S., & Weisz, J. R. (2017). Amelioration of child depression through behavioral parent training: A preliminary study. *Journal of Clinical Child and Adolescent Psychology, 46*(4), 611–618. https://doi.org/10.1080/15374416.2015.1050722

Edwards, V. J., Holden, G. W., Felitti, V. J., & Anda, R. F. (2003). Relationship between multiple forms of childhood maltreatment and adult mental health in community respondents: Results from the adverse childhood experiences study. *American Journal of Psychiatry, 160*(8), 1453–1460. https://doi.org/10.1176/appi.ajp.160.8.1453

Eells, T. D. (2015). *Psychotherapy case formulation.* American Psychological Association. https://doi.org/10.1037/14667-000

Ehlers, A., & Clark, D. M. (2000). A cognitive model of posttraumatic stress disorder. *Behaviour Research and Therapy, 38*(4), 319–345. https://doi.org/10.1016/S0005-7967(99)00123-0

Ehlers, A., Mayou, R. A., & Bryant, B. (2003). Cognitive predictors of posttraumatic stress disorder in children: Results of a prospective longitudinal study. *Behaviour Research and Therapy, 41*(1), 1–10. https://doi.org/10.1016/s0005-7967(01)00126-7

Eisenberg, N., Spinrad, T. L., & Eggum, N. D. (2010). Emotion-related self-regulation and its relation to children's maladjustment. *Annual Review of Clinical Psychology, 6*, 495–525. https://doi.org/10.1146/annurev.clinpsy.121208.131208

Ekhtiari, H., Rezapour, T., Aupperle, R. L., & Paulus, M. P. (2017). Neuroscience-informed psychoeducation for addiction medicine: A neurocognitive perspective. *Progress in Brain Research, 235*, 239–264. https://doi.org/10.1016/bs.pbr.2017.08.013

Engel, G. L. (1977). The need for a new medical model: A challenge for biomedicine. *Science, 196*(4286), 129–136. https://doi.org/10.1126/science.847460

Engel, G. L. (1980). The clinical application of the biopsychosocial model. *The American Journal of Psychiatry, 137*(5), 535–544. https://doi.org/10.1176/ajp.137.5.535

Epstein, M. H., Mooney, P., Ryser, G., & Pierce, C. D. (2004). Validity and reliability of the behavioral and emotional rating scale (2nd edition): Youth rating scale. *Research on Social Work Practice, 14*(5), 358–367. https://doi.org/10.1177/1049731504265832

Erichsen, J. (1866). *On railway and other injuries of the nervous system*. Walton and Moberly.

Erk, R. R. (Ed.) (2008). *Counseling treatment for children and adolescents with DSM-IV-TR disorders* (2nd ed.). Pearson/Merrill Prentice Hall.

Eulenberg, A. (1878). *Lehrbuch der Nervenkrankheiten [Textbook in Neurological Diseases]*. August Hirschwald.

Falender, C. A., & Shafranske, E. P. (2012). *Getting the most out of clinical training and supervision: A guide for practicum students and interns* (1st ed.). American Psychological Association.

Felitti, V. J., Anda, R. F., Nordenberg, D., Williamson, D. F., Spitz, A. M., Edwards, V., Koss, M. P., & Marks, J. S. (1998). Relationship of childhood abuse and household dysfunction to many of the leading causes of death in adults. The Adverse Childhood Experiences (ACE) Study. *American Journal of Preventive Medicine, 14*(4), 245–258. https://doi.org/10.1016/S0749-3797(98)00017-8

Fergusson, D. M., Horwood, L. J., & Lynskey, M. T. (1996). Childhood sexual abuse and psychiatric disorder in young adulthood: II. Psychiatric outcomes of childhood sexual abuse. *Journal of the American Academy of Child & Adolescent Psychiatry, 35*(10), 1365–1374. https://doi.org/10.1097/00004583-199610000-00024

Fergusson, D. M., & Lynskey, M. T. (1997). Physical punishment/maltreatment during childhood and adjustment in young adulthood. *Child Abuse & Neglect, 21*(7), 617–630. https://doi.org/10.1016/S0145-2134(97)00021-5

Figley, C. (1978). *Stress disorders among Vietnam veterans: Theory, research and treatment*. Routledge.

Finkelhor, D., Ormrod, R. K., & Turner, H. A. (2007). Poly-victimization: A neglected component in child victimization. *Child Abuse & Neglect, 31*(1), 7–26. https://doi.org/10.1016/j.chiabu.2006.06.008

Finkelhor, D., Ormrod, R. K., & Turner, H. A. (2009). The developmental epidemiology of childhood victimization. *Journal of Interpersonal Violence, 24*(5), 711–731. https://doi.org/10.1177/0886260508317185

Finkelhor, D., Shattuck, A., Turner, H., & Hamby, S. (2015a). A revised inventory of adverse childhood experiences. *Child Abuse & Neglect, 48*, 13–21. https://doi.org/10.1016/j.chiabu.2015.07.011

Finkelhor, D., Turner, H. A., Shattuck, A., & Hamby, S. L. (2015b). Prevalence of childhood exposure to violence, crime, and abuse: Results from the national survey of children's exposure to violence. *JAMA Pediatrics, 169*(8), 746. https://doi.org/10.1001/jamapediatrics.2015.0676

Flaherty, E. G., Thompson, R., Dubowitz, H., Harvey, E. M., English, D. J., Proctor, L. J., & Runyan, D. K. (2013). Adverse childhood experiences and child health in early adolescence. *JAMA Pediatrics, 167*(7), 622. https://doi.org/10.1001/jamapediatrics.2013.22

Fletcher, K. (1996a). Psychometric review of the childhood PTSD interview. In B. H. Stamm (Ed.), *Measurement of stress, trauma, and adaptation* (pp. 87–89). Sidran Press.

Fletcher, K. (1996b). Psychometric review of the parent report of child's reaction to stress. In B. H. Stamm (Ed.), *Measurement of stress, trauma, and adaptation* (pp. 225–227). Sidran Press.

Foa, E. B., Asnaani, A., Zang, Y., Capaldi, S., & Yeh, R. (2018). Psychometrics of the child PTSD symptom scale for DSM-5 for trauma-exposed children and adolescents. *Journal of Clinical Child & Adolescent Psychology, 47*(1), 38–46. https://doi.org/10.1080/15374416.2017.1350962

Ford, J. D., Grasso, D., Greene, C., Levine, J., Spinazzola, J., & van der Kolk, B. (2013). Clinical significance of a proposed developmental trauma disorder diagnosis: Results of an international survey of clinicians. *The Journal of Clinical Psychiatry, 74*(8), 841–849. https://doi.org/10.4088/JCP.12m08030

Ford, J. D., Spinazzola, J., van der Kolk, B., & Grasso, D. J. (2018). Toward an empirically based developmental trauma disorder diagnosis for children: Factor structure, item characteristics, reliability, and validity of the developmental trauma disorder semi-structured interview. *The Journal of Clinical Psychiatry, 79*(5), 17m11675. https://doi.org/10.4088/JCP.17m11675

Forde, A. T., Crookes, D. M., Suglia, S. F., & Demmer, R. T. (2019). The weathering hypothesis as an explanation for racial disparities in health: A systematic review. *Annals of Epidemiology, 33*, 1–18.e3. https://doi.org/10.1016/j.annepidem.2019.02.011

Frederick, C., Pynoos, R. S., & Nader, K. (1992). *Child post-traumatic stress disorder reaction index (CPTSD-RI)*. Department of Psychiatry, University of California, Los Angeles.

Freud, S. (1959). *The collected papers*. Basic Books.

Galano, M. M., & Graham-Bermann, S. A. (2019). Traumatic stress within the family. In B. H. Fiese, M. Celano, K. Deater-Deckard, E. N. Jouriles, & M. A. Whisman (Eds.), *APA handbook of contemporary family psychology: Applications and broad impact of family psychology* (Vol. 2, pp. 539–554). American Psychological Association. https://doi.org/10.1037/0000100-033

Galea, S. (2021, May 20). Why health? *The Healthiest Goldfish*. https://sandrogalea.substack.com/p/why-health?utm_source=url

Gelles, R. J., & Maynard, P. E. (1987). A structural family systems approach to intervention in cases of family violence. *Family Relations*, *36*(3), 270. https://doi .org/10.2307/583539

Geronimus, A. T., Hicken, M., Keene, D., & Bound, J. (2006). "Weathering" and age patterns of allostatic load scores among blacks and whites in the United States. *American Journal of Public Health*, *96*(5), 826–833. https://doi.org/10 .2105/AJPH.2004.060749

Gioia, G. A., Isquith, P. K., Retzlaff, P. D., & Espy, K. A. (2002). Confirmatory factor analysis of the behavior rating inventory of executive function (BRIEF) in a clinical sample. *Child Neuropsychology*, *8*(4), 249–257. https://doi.org/10 .1076/chin.8.4.249.13513

Giola, G., Isquith, P., Guy, S., & Kenworthy, L. (2000). *Behavior rating inventory of executive function: Professional manual*. Psychological Assessment Resources.

Gonzalez, M. A., & Jones, D. J. (2016). Cascading effects of BPT for child internalizing problems and caregiver depression. *Clinical Psychology Review*, *50*, 11–21. https://doi.org/10.1016/j.cpr.2016.09.007

Goodman, G. S., Quas, J. A., & Ogle, C. M. (2010). Child maltreatment and memory. *Annual Review of Psychology*, *61*(1), 325–351. https://doi.org/10.1146/ annurev.psych.093008.100403

Grasso, D. J., Dierkhising, C. B., Branson, C. E., Ford, J. D., & Lee, R. (2016). Developmental patterns of adverse childhood experiences and current symptoms and impairment in youth referred for trauma-specific services. *Journal of Abnormal Child Psychology*, *44*(5), 871–886. https://doi.org/10.1007/ s10802-015-0086-8

Green, A. H. (1988). Child maltreatment and its victims. A comparison of physical and sexual abuse. *The Psychiatric Clinics of North America*, *11*(4), 591–610. https://doi.org/10.1016/S0193-953X(18)30472-6

Greene, C. A., Chan, G., McCarthy, K. J., Wakschlag, L. S., & Briggs-Gowan, M. J. (2018). Psychological and physical intimate partner violence and young children's mental health: The role of maternal posttraumatic stress symptoms and parenting behaviors. *Child Abuse & Neglect*, *77*, 168–179. https://doi.org/ 10.1016/j.chiabu.2018.01.012

Grinker, R., & Spiegel, J. (1945). *Men under stress*. McGraw-Hill.

Gross, J. J. (1998). The emerging field of emotion regulation: An integrative review. *Review of General Psychology*, *2*(3), 271–299. https://doi.org/10.1037/ 1089-2680.2.3.271

Gross, J. J., & Barrett, L. F. (2011). Emotion generation and emotion regulation: One or two depends on your point of view. *Emotion Review: Journal of the International Society for Research on Emotion*, *3*(1), 8–16. https://doi.org/10 .1177/1754073910380974

Hadaway, S. M., & Brue, A. W. (2016). *Practitioner's guide to functional behavioral assessment*. Springer International Publishing. https://doi.org/10.1007/978-3- 319-23721-3

Hannesdóttir, D. K., & Ollendick, T. H. (2017). Emotion regulation and anxiety: Developmental psychopathology and treatment. In C. A. Essau, S. LeBlanc, & T. H. Ollendick (Eds.), *Emotion regulation and psychopathology in children and adolescents.* (pp. 154–170). Oxford University Press.

Hartvig, P. (1977). Krigsseilersyndromet [The war sailor syndrome]. *Nordisk Psykiatrisk Tidsskrift, 29,* 302–313.

Heleniak, C., Jenness, J. L., Vander Stoep, A., McCauley, E., & McLaughlin, K. A. (2016). Childhood maltreatment exposure and disruptions in emotion regulation: A transdiagnostic pathway to adolescent internalizing and externalizing psychopathology. *Cognitive Therapy and Research, 40*(3), 394–415. https://doi.org/10.1007/s10608-015-9735-z

Hermann, K., & Thygesen, P. (1954). Kz syndromet [The concentration camp syndrome]. *Ugeskrift for Laeger, 116,* 825–836.

Hesnard, A. (1914). Les troubles nerveux et psychiques consecutifs aux catastrophes navales [Mental and nervous symptoms following naval disasters]. *Revue de Psychiatrie, 18,* 139–151.

Hickman, L. J., Jaycox, L. H., Setodji, C. M., Kofner, A., Schultz, D., Barnes-Proby, D., & Harris, R. (2013). How much does "how much" matter? Assessing the relationship between children's lifetime exposure to violence and trauma symptoms, behavior problems, and parenting stress. *Journal of Interpersonal Violence, 28*(6), 1338–1362. https://doi.org/10.1177/0886260512468239

Higa-McMillan, C. K., Francis, S. E., Rith-Najarian, L., & Chorpita, B. F. (2016). Evidence base update: 50 years of research on treatment for child and adolescent anxiety. *Journal of Clinical Child and Adolescent Psychology: The Official Journal for the Society of Clinical Child and Adolescent Psychology, American Psychological Association, Division 53, 45*(2), 91–113. https://doi.org/10.1080/15374416.2015.1046177

Hodges, K., Doucette-Gates, A., & Kim, C. S. (2000). Predicting service utilization with the Child and Adolescent Functional Assessment Scale in a sample of youths with serious emotional disturbance served by center for mental health services-funded demonstrations. *The Journal of Behavioral Health Services & Research, 27*(1), 47–59. https://doi.org/10.1007/BF02287803

Hodges, K., Doucette-Gates, A., & Liao, Q. (1999). The relationship between the child and adolescent functional assessment scale (CAFAS) and indicators of functioning. *Journal of Child and Family Studies, 8*(1), 109–122. https://doi.org/10.1023/A:1022902812761

Hodges, K., & Gust, J. (1995). Measures of impairment for children and adolescents. *Journal of Mental Health Administration, 22*(4), 403–413. https://doi.org/10.1007/BF02518634

Hodges, K., & Kim, C. S. (2000). Psychometric study of the child and adolescent functional assessment scale: Prediction of contact with the law and poor school attendance. *Journal of Abnormal Child Psychology, 28*(3), 287–297. https://doi.org/10.1023/a:1005100521818

Hodges, K., & Wong, M. M. (1996). Psychometric characteristics of a multidimensional measure to assess impairment: The child and adolescent functional assessment scale. *Journal of Child and Family Studies, 5*(4), 445–467. https://doi.org/10.1007/BF02233865

Hodges, K., Wong, M. M., & Latessa, M. (1998). Use of the child and adolescent functional assessment scale (CAFAS) as an outcome measure in clinical settings. *The Journal of Behavioral Health Services & Research, 25*(3), 325–336. https://doi.org/10.1007/BF02287471

Hodges, K., Wotring, J., Forgatch, M. S., Lyon, A., & Spangler, J. (2008). Outcome indicators for youth's functioning and parent's child management skills: Results from PMTO training. In *The 21st Annual Research Conference Proceedings* (pp. 55–56). http://rtckids.fmhi.usf.edu/rtcconference/21stconference/agenda/21Agenda.pdf

Howe, M. L., Cicchetti, D., & Toth, S. L. (2006). Children's basic memory processes, stress, and maltreatment. *Development and Psychopathology, 18*(03). https://doi.org/10.1017/S0954579406060378

Howes, P. W., Cicchetti, D., Toth, S. L., & Rogosch, F. A. (2000). Affective, organizational, and relational characteristics of maltreating families: A system's perspective. *Journal of Family Psychology, 14*(1), 95–110. https://doi.org/10.1037/0893-3200.14.1.95

Jaycox, L. (2004). *CBITS: Cognitive behavioral intervention for trauma in schools.* Sopris West Educational Services.

Jensen, T., Cohen, J., Jaycox, L., & Rosner, R. (2020). Treatment of PTSD and complex PTSD. In D. Forbes, J. I. Bisson, C. M. Monson, & L. Berliner (Eds.), *Effective treatments for PTSD: Practice guidelines from the international society for traumatic stress studies* (3rd ed., 2pp. 385–413). The Guilford Press.

Jiang, S., Postovit, L., Cattaneo, A., Binder, E. B., & Aitchison, K. J. (2019). Epigenetic modifications in stress response genes associated with childhood trauma. *Frontiers in Psychiatry, 10*, 808. https://doi.org/10.3389/fpsyt.2019.00808

Jones, C. P. (2001). Invited commentary: "race," racism, and the practice of epidemiology. *American Journal of Epidemiology, 154*(4), 299–304; discussion 305-306. https://doi.org/10.1093/aje/154.4.299

Jongsma, A. E., Peterson, L. M., McInnis, W. P., & Bruce, T. J. (2014). *The child psychotherapy treatment planner* (5th ed.). Wiley.

Jud, A., Fallon, B., & Trocmé, N. (2012). Who gets services and who does not? Multi-level approach to the decision for ongoing child welfare or referral to specialized services. *Children and Youth Services Review, 34*(5), 983–988. https://doi.org/10.1016/j.childyouth.2012.01.030

Kaplow, J. B., Rolon-Arroyo, B., Layne, C. M., Rooney, E., Oosterhoff, B., Hill, R., Steinberg, A. M., Lotterman, J., Gallagher, K. A. S., & Pynoos, R. S. (2020). Validation of the UCLA PTSD reaction index for DSM-5: A developmentally informed assessment tool for youth. *Journal of the American Academy of Child*

& *Adolescent Psychiatry*, 59(1), 186–194. https://doi.org/10.1016/j.jaac.2018.10.019

Kardiner, A. (1941). *The traumatic neuroses of war*. Aronson.

Kassam-Adams, N. (2006). The acute stress checklist for children (ASC-Kids): Development of a child self-report measure. *Journal of Traumatic Stress*, 19(1), 129–139. https://doi.org/10.1002/jts.20090

Kaufman, J., Birmaher, B., Brent, D., Rao, U., Flynn, C., Moreci, P., Williamson, D., & Ryan, N. (1997). Schedule for affective disorders and schizophrenia for school-age children-present and lifetime version (K-SADS-PL): Initial reliability and validity data. *Journal of the American Academy of Child & Adolescent Psychiatry*, 36(7), 980–988. https://doi.org/10.1097/00004583-199707000-00021

Kaufman, J., & Cicchetti, D. (1989). Effects of maltreatment on school-age children's socioemotional development: Assessments in a day-camp setting. *Developmental Psychology*, 25(4), 516–524. https://doi.org/10.1037/0012-1649.25.4.516

Kavanaugh, B., & Holler, K. (2015). Brief report: Neurocognitive functioning in adolescents following childhood maltreatment and evidence for underlying planning & organizational deficits. *Child Neuropsychology*, 21(6), 840–848. https://doi.org/10.1080/09297049.2014.929101

Kavanaugh, B. C., Dupont-Frechette, J. A., Jerskey, B. A., & Holler, K. A. (2017). Neurocognitive deficits in children and adolescents following maltreatment: Neurodevelopmental consequences and neuropsychological implications of traumatic stress. *Applied Neuropsychology: Child*, 6(1), 64–78. https://doi.org/10.1080/21622965.2015.1079712

Kazak, A. E., Alderfer, M., Enlow, P. T., Lewis, A. M., Vega, G., Barakat, L., Kassam-Adams, N., Pai, A., Canter, K. S., Hildenbrand, A. K., McDonnell, G. A., Price, J., Schultz, C., Sood, E., & Phan, T.-L. (2021). COVID-19 exposure and family impact scales: Factor structure and initial psychometrics. *Journal of Pediatric Psychology*, 46(5), 504–513. https://doi.org/10.1093/jpepsy/jsab026

Kazdin, A. E. (2005). *Parent management training: Treatment for oppositional, aggressive, and antisocial behavior in children and adolescents*. Oxford University Press.

Kazdin, A. E., Siegel, T. C., & Bass, D. (1992). Cognitive problem-solving skills training and parent management training in the treatment of antisocial behavior in children. *Journal of Consulting and Clinical Psychology*, 60(5), 733–747. https://doi.org/10.1037/0022-006X.60.5.733

Kazdin, A. E., & Whitley, M. K. (2003). Treatment of parental stress to enhance therapeutic change among children referred for aggressive and antisocial behavior. *Journal of Consulting and Clinical Psychology*, 71(3), 504–515. http://imagesrvr.epnet.com/embimages/pdh2/ccp/ccp713504.pdf

Keiley, M. K., Howe, T. R., Dodge, K. A., Bates, J. E., & Petti, G. S. (2001). The timing of child physical maltreatment: A cross-domain growth analysis of impact on adolescent externalizing and internalizing problems. *Development and Psychopathology, 13*(4), 891–912. https://doi.org/10.1017/S0954579401004084

Keller, S. M., Burton, M. S., & Feeny, N. (2017). Posttraumatic stress disorder in youth. In C. Flessner & J. Piacentini (Eds.), *The clinical handbook of psychological disorders in children and adolescents: A step-by-step treatment manual* (pp. 240–272). Guilford Press.

Kempe, C. H. (1962). The battered-child syndrome. *JAMA: The Journal of the American Medical Association, 181*(1), 17. https://doi.org/10.1001/jama.1962.03050270019004

Kenardy, J. A., Spence, S. H., & Macleod, A. C. (2006). Screening for posttraumatic stress disorder in children after accidental injury. *Pediatrics, 118*(3), 1002–1009. https://doi.org/10.1542/peds.2006-0406

Kendall-Tackett, K. A., & Eckenrode, J. (1996). The effects of neglect on academic achievement and disciplinary problems: A developmental perspective. *Child Abuse & Neglect, 20*(3), 161–169. https://doi.org/10.1016/S0145-2134(95)00139-5

Kilpatrick, D. G., Ruggiero, K. J., Acierno, R., Saunders, B. E., Resnick, H. S., & Best, C. L. (2003). Violence and risk of PTSD, major depression, substance abuse/dependence, and comorbidity: Results from the National Survey of Adolescents. *Journal of Consulting and Clinical Psychology, 71*(4), 692–700. https://doi.org/10.1037/0022-006X.71.4.692

Kim, J., & Cicchetti, D. (2010). Longitudinal pathways linking child maltreatment, emotion regulation, peer relations, and psychopathology. *Journal of Child Psychology and Psychiatry, and Allied Disciplines, 51*(6), 706–716. https://doi.org/10.1111/j.1469-7610.2009.02202.x

Kiser, L. J., Stover, C. S., Navalta, C. P., Dorado, J., Vogel, J. M., Abdul-Adil, J. K., Kim, S., Lee, R. C., Vivrette, R., & Briggs, E. C. (2014). Effects of the child–perpetrator relationship on mental health outcomes of child abuse: It's (not) all relative. *Child Abuse & Neglect, 38*(6), 1083–1093. https://doi.org/10.1016/j.chiabu.2014.02.017

Kotch, J. B., Lewis, T., Hussey, J. M., English, D., Thompson, R., Litrownik, A. J., Runyan, D. K., Bangdiwala, S. I., Margolis, B., & Dubowitz, H. (2008). Importance of early neglect for childhood aggression. *Pediatrics, 121*(4), 725–731. https://doi.org/10.1542/peds.2006-3622

La Greca, A., Silverman, W. K., Vernberg, E. M., & Prinstein, M. J. (1996). Symptoms of posttraumatic stress in children after Hurricane Andrew: A prospective study. *Journal of Consulting and Clinical Psychology, 64*(4), 712–723. https://doi.org/10.1037//0022-006x.64.4.712

Landes, S. J. (2019). Conducting effective behavioural and solution analyses. In M. A. Swales (Ed.), *The Oxford handbook of dialectical behaviour therapy.* (pp. 259–282). Oxford University Press.

Lane, R. D., Quinlan, D. M., Schwartz, G. E., Walker, P. A., & Zeitlin, S. (1990). The levels of emotional awareness scale: A cognitive-developmental measure of emotion. *Journal of Personality Assessment, 55*(1–2), 124–134. https://doi.org/10.1207/s15327752jpa5501&2_12

Lang, J., McKie, J., Smith, H., McLaughlin, A., Gillberg, C., Shiels, P. G., & Minnis, H. (2020). Adverse childhood experiences, epigenetics and telomere length variation in childhood and beyond: A systematic review of the literature. *European Child & Adolescent Psychiatry, 29*(10), 1329–1338. https://doi.org/10.1007/s00787-019-01329-1

Lang, J. M., & Connell, C. M. (2017). Development and validation of a brief trauma screening measure for children: The child trauma screen. *Psychological Trauma: Theory, Research, Practice, and Policy, 9*(3), 390–398. https://doi.org/10.1037/tra0000235

Lansford, J. E., Dodge, K. A., Pettit, G. S., Bates, J. E., Crozier, J., & Kaplow, J. (2002). A 12-year prospective study of the long-term effects of early child physical maltreatment on psychological, behavioral, and academic problems in adolescence. *Archives of Pediatrics & Adolescent Medicine, 156*(8), 824–830. https://doi.org/10.1001/archpedi.156.8.824

Layne, C. M., Greeson, J. K. P., Ostrowski, S. A., Kim, S., Reading, S., Vivrette, R. L., Briggs, E. C., Fairbank, J. A., & Pynoos, R. S. (2014). Cumulative trauma exposure and high risk behavior in adolescence: Findings from the l child traumatic stress network core data set. *Psychological Trauma: Theory, Research, Practice, and Policy, 6*(Suppl 1), S40–S49. https://doi.org/10.1037/a0037799

Layne, C. M., Kaplow, J. B., & Youngstrom, E. A. (2017). Applying evidence-based assessment to childhood trauma and bereavement: Concepts, principles, and practices. In M. A. Landolt, M. Cloitre, & U. Schnyder (Eds.), *Evidence-based treatments for trauma related disorders in children and adolescents* (pp. 67–96). Springer International Publishing. https://doi.org/10.1007/978-3-319-46138-0_4

Lee, R. T., Perez, A. D., Boykin, C. M., & Mendoza-Denton, R. (2019). On the prevalence of racial discrimination in the United States. *PLOS ONE, 14*(1), e0210698. https://doi.org/10.1371/journal.pone.0210698

Lehman, B. J., David, D. M., & Gruber, J. A. (2017). Rethinking the biopsychosocial model of health: Understanding health as a dynamic system. *Social and Personality Psychology Compass, 11*(8), e12328. https://doi.org/10.1111/spc3.12328

Leiter, J., & Johnsen, M. C. (1994). Child maltreatment and school performance. *American Journal of Education, 102*(2), 154–189. https://doi.org/10.1086/444063

Leiter, J., & Johnsen, M. C. (1997). Child Maltreatment and school performance declines: An event-history analysis. *American Educational Research Journal, 34*(3), 563–589. https://doi.org/10.3102/00028312034003563

Lewis, S. J., Arseneault, L., Caspi, A., Fisher, H. L., Matthews, T., Moffitt, T. E., Odgers, C. L., Stahl, D., Teng, J. Y., & Danese, A. (2019). The epidemiology of trauma and post-traumatic stress disorder in a representative cohort of young people in England and Wales. *The Lancet. Psychiatry, 6*(3), 247–256. https://doi .org/10.1016/S2215-0366(19)30031-8

Lewis-Fernández, R., Aggarwal, N. K., Hinton, L., Hinton, D. E., & Kirmayer, L. J. (2016). *DSM-5® handbook on the cultural formulation interview.* (R. Lewis-Fernández, N. K. Aggarwal, L. Hinton, D. E. Hinton, & L. J. Kirmayer (Eds.)). American Psychiatric Publishing, Inc.

Lippard, E. T. C., & Nemeroff, C. B. (2020). The devastating clinical consequences of child abuse and neglect: Increased disease vulnerability and poor treatment response in mood disorders. *American Journal of Psychiatry, 177*(1), 20–36. https://doi.org/10.1176/appi.ajp.2019.19010020

Lynch, M., & Cicchetti, D. (1998). An ecological-transactional analysis of children and contexts: The longitudinal interplay among child maltreatment, community violence, and children's symptomatology. *Development and Psychopathology, 10*(2), 235–257. https://doi.org/10.1017/S095457949800159X

Lynch, M. A. (1985). Child abuse before Kempe: An historical literature review. *Child Abuse & Neglect, 9*(1), 7–15. https://doi.org/10.1016/0145-2134(85)90086-9

Malinosky-Rummell, R., & Hansen, D. J. (1993). Long-term consequences of childhood physical abuse. *Psychological Bulletin, 114*(1), 68–79. https://doi.org/10.1037/0033-2909.114.1.68

Manly, J. T., Kim, J. E., Rogosch, F. A., & Cicchetti, D. (2001). Dimensions of child maltreatment and children's adjustment: Contributions of developmental timing and subtype. *Development and Psychopathology, 13*(4), 759–782.

Manzoni, M., Fernandez, I., Bertella, S., Tizzoni, F., Gazzola, E., Molteni, M., & Nobile, M. (2021). Eye movement desensitization and reprocessing: The state of the art of efficacy in children and adolescent with post traumatic stress disorder. *Journal of Affective Disorders, 282*, 340–347. https://doi.org/10.1016/j .jad.2020.12.088

Marchette, L. K., & Weisz, J. R. (2017). Practitioner review: Empirical evolution of youth psychotherapy toward transdiagnostic approaches. *Journal of Child Psychology and Psychiatry, 58*(9), 970–984. https://doi.org/10.1111/jcpp.12747

Martin, R. E., & Ochsner, K. N. (2016). The neuroscience of emotion regulation development: Implications for education. *Current Opinion in Behavioral Sciences, 10*, 142–148. https://doi.org/10.1016/j.cobeha.2016.06.006

Masten, A. S., & Barnes, A. J. (2018). Resilience in children: Developmental perspectives. *Children (Basel, Switzerland), 5*(7), E98. https://doi.org/10.3390/ children5070098

Maughan, A., & Cicchetti, D. (2002). Impact of child maltreatment and interadult violence on children's emotion regulation abilities and socioemotional adjustment. *Child Development*, *73*(5), 1525–1542. https://doi.org/10.1111/1467-8624.00488

Mays, V. M., Cochran, S. D., & Barnes, N. W. (2007). Race, race-based discrimination, and health outcomes among African Americans. *Annual Review of Psychology*, *58*, 201–225. https://doi.org/10.1146/annurev.psych.57.102904.190212

McEwen, B. S. (2006). Protective and damaging effects of stress mediators: Central role of the brain. *Dialogues in Clinical Neuroscience*, *8*(4), 367–381.

McEwen, C. A., & Gregerson, S. F. (2019). A critical assessment of the adverse childhood experiences study at 20 years. *American Journal of Preventive Medicine*, *56*(6), 790–794. https://doi.org/10.1016/j.amepre.2018.10.016

McLaughlin, K. A. (2016). Future directions in childhood adversity and youth psychopathology. *Journal of Clinical Child & Adolescent Psychology*, *45*(3), 361–382. https://doi.org/10.1080/15374416.2015.1110823

McLaughlin, K. A., Busso, D. S., Duys, A., Green, J. G., Alves, S., Way, M., & Sheridan, M. A. (2014). Amygdala response to negative stimuli predicts PTSD symptom onset following a terrorist attack. *Depression and Anxiety*, *31*(10), 834–842. https://doi.org/10.1002/da.22284

McLaughlin, K. A., Peverill, M., Gold, A. L., Alves, S., & Sheridan, M. A. (2015). Child maltreatment and neural systems underlying emotion regulation. *Journal of the American Academy of Child and Adolescent Psychiatry*, *54*(9), 753–762. https://doi.org/10.1016/j.jaac.2015.06.010

Meiser-Stedman, R., Smith, P., Bryant, R., Salmon, K., Yule, W., Dalgleish, T., & Nixon, R. D. V. (2009). Development and validation of the child post-traumatic cognitions inventory (CPTCI). *Journal of Child Psychology and Psychiatry*, *50*(4), 432–440. https://doi.org/10.1111/j.1469-7610.2008.01995.x

Meyer, I. H. (2003). Prejudice as stress: Conceptual and measurement problems. *American Journal of Public Health*, *93*(2), 262–265. https://doi.org/10.2105/ajph.93.2.262

Mooney, P., Epstein, M. H., Ryser, G., & Pierce, C. D. (2005). Reliability and validity of the behavioral and emotional rating scale-second edition: Parent rating scale. *Children & Schools*, *27*(3), 147–155. https://doi.org/10.1093/cs/27.3.147

Motlova, L. B., Balon, R., Beresin, E. V., Brenner, A. M., Coverdale, J. H., Guerrero, A. P. S., Louie, A. K., & Roberts, L. W. (2017). Psychoeducation as an opportunity for patients, psychiatrists, and psychiatric educators: Why do we ignore it? *Academic Psychiatry*, *41*(4), 447–451. https://doi.org/10.1007/s40596-017-0728-y

Myers, C. (1915). A contribution to the study of shell shock. *Lancet*, *1*, 316–320.

Myers, C. (1940). *Shell shock in France 1914–1918*. Cambridge University Press.

National Center for Study of Corporal Punishment and Alternatives in Schools. (1992). *My worst experiences survey*. Temple University Press.

Navalta, C. P. (2011). Neuropsychological aspects of child abuse and neglect. In A. S. Davis (Ed.), *Handbook of pediatric neuropsychology* (pp. 1039–1050). Springer Publishing Co.

Navalta, C. P., Ashy, M., & Teicher, M. (2008a). Emotional trauma. In G. Reyes, J. D. Elhai, & J. D. Ford (Eds.), *Encyclopedia of psychological trauma* (pp. 246–249). John Wiley & Sons.

Navalta, C. P., Brown, A. D., Nisewaner, A., Ellis, B. H., & Saxe, G. N. (2013). Trauma systems therapy. In J. D. Ford & C. A. Courtois (Eds.), *Treating complex traumatic stress disorders in children and adolescents: Scientific foundations and therapeutic models.* (pp. 329–347). Guilford Press.

Navalta, C. P., & Moore, A. (2016, November). A recipe for case conceptualization: Understanding clients at the intersection of science and art. *The Advocate Magazine, 39*(4), 10–12.

Navalta, C. P., Polcari, A., Webster, D. M., Boghossian, A., & Teicher, M. H. (2006). Effects of childhood sexual abuse on neuropsychological and cognitive function in college women. *The Journal of Neuropsychiatry and Clinical Neurosciences, 18*(1), 45–53. https://doi.org/10.1176/jnp.18.1.45

Navalta, C. P., Tomoda, A., & Teicher, M. H. (2008b). Trajectories of neuro-behavioral development: The clinical neuroscience of child abuse. In M. L. Howe, G. S. Goodman, & D. Cicchetti (Eds.), *Stress, trauma, and children's memory development: Neurobiological, cognitive, clinical, and legal perspectives* (pp. 50–82). Oxford University Press. https://doi.org/10.1093/acprof:oso/9780195308457.003.0003

NCTSN Core Curriculum on Childhood Trauma Task Force. (2012). *The 12 core concepts: Concepts for understanding traumatic stress responses in children and families. Core curriculum on childhood trauma.* UCLA-Duke University National Center for Child Traumatic Stress.

Nemeroff, C. B. (2016). Paradise lost: The neurobiological and clinical consequences of child abuse and neglect. *Neuron, 89*(5), 892–909. https://doi.org/10.1016/j.neuron.2016.01.019

Nolin, P., & Ethier, L. (2007). Using neuropsychological profiles to classify neglected children with or without physical abuse. *Child Abuse & Neglect, 31*(6), 631–643. https://doi.org/10.1016/j.chiabu.2006.12.009

Oral, R., Ramirez, M., Coohey, C., Nakada, S., Walz, A., Kuntz, A., Benoit, J., & Peek-Asa, C. (2016). Adverse childhood experiences and trauma informed care: The future of health care. *Pediatric Research, 79*(1–2), 227–233. https://doi.org/10.1038/pr.2015.197

Pachter, L. M., & Coll, C. G. (2009). Racism and child health: A review of the literature and future directions. *Journal of Developmental & Behavioral Pediatrics, 30*(3), 255–263. https://doi.org/10.1097/DBP.0b013e3181a7ed5a

Pachter, L. M., Szalacha, L. A., Bernstein, B. A., & García Coll, C. (2010). Perceptions of racism in children and youth (PRaCY): Properties of a self-report instrument for research on children's health and development. *Ethnicity & Health, 15*(1), 33–46. https://doi.org/10.1080/13557850903383196

Page, H. (1883). *Injuries of the spine and spinal cord without apparent mechanical lesion and nervous shock in their surgical and medicolegal aspects.* Churchill.

Paradies, Y., Ben, J., Denson, N., Elias, A., Priest, N., Pieterse, A., Gupta, A., Kelaher, M., & Gee, G. (2015). Racism as a determinant of health: A systematic review and meta-analysis. *PLOS ONE, 10*(9), e0138511. https://doi.org/10.1371/journal.pone.0138511

Paradies, Y. C. (2006). Defining, conceptualizing and characterizing racism in health research. *Critical Public Health, 16*(2), 143–157. https://doi.org/10.1080/09581590600828881

Patrick, S. W., Henkhaus, L. E., Zickafoose, J. S., Lovell, K., Halvorson, A., Loch, S., Letterie, M., & Davis, M. M. (2020). Well-being of parents and children during the COVID-19 pandemic: A national survey. *Pediatrics, 146*(4), e2020016824. https://doi.org/10.1542/peds.2020-016824

Patterson, J. M. (1991). A family systems perspective for working with youth with disability. *Pediatrician, 18*(2), 129–141.

Perrin, S., Meiser-Stedman, R., & Smith, P. (2005). The children's revised impact of event scale (CRIES): Validity as a screening instrument for PTSD. *Behavioural and Cognitive Psychotherapy, 33*(4), 487–498. https://doi.org/10.1017/S1352465805002419

Phelps, C., & Sperry, L. L. (2020). Children and the COVID-19 pandemic. *Psychological Trauma: Theory, Research, Practice and Policy, 12*(S1), S73–S75. https://doi.org/10.1037/tra0000861

Pollak, S. D. (2015). Multilevel developmental approaches to understanding the effects of child maltreatment: Recent advances and future challenges. *Development and Psychopathology, 27*(4 Pt 2), 1387–1397. https://doi.org/10.1017/S0954579415000826

Pollak, S. D., Vardi, S., Putzer Bechner, A. M., & Curtin, J. J. (2005). Physically abused children's regulation of attention in response to hostility. *Child Development, 76*(5), 968–977. https://doi.org/10.1111/j.1467-8624.2005.00890.x

Poznanski, J. J., & McLennan, J. (1995). Conceptualizing and measuring counselors' theoretical orientation. *Journal of Counseling Psychology, 42*(4), 411–422. https://doi.org/10.1037/0022-0167.42.4.411

Priest, N., Paradies, Y., Trenerry, B., Truong, M., Karlsen, S., & Kelly, Y. (2013). A systematic review of studies examining the relationship between reported racism and health and wellbeing for children and young people. *Social Science & Medicine, 95*, 115–127. https://doi.org/10.1016/j.socscimed.2012.11.031

Prochaska, J. O., & DiClemente, C. C. (1983). Stages and processes of self-change of smoking: Toward an integrative model of change. *Journal of Consulting and Clinical Psychology, 51*(3), 390–395. https://doi.org/10.1037/0022-006X.51.3.390

Proctor, L. J., Lewis, T., Roesch, S., Thompson, R., Litrownik, A. J., English, D., Arria, A. M., Isbell, P., & Dubowitz, H. (2017). Child maltreatment and age of alcohol and marijuana initiation in high-risk youth. *Addictive Behaviors, 75,* 64–69. https://doi.org/10.1016/j.addbeh.2017.06.021

Putnam, F. W., Harris, W. W., Lieberman, A., Putnam, K. T., & Amaya-Jackson, L. (2015). *Childhood adversity narratives.* CANarratives.org.

Putnam, K. T., Harris, W. W., & Putnam, F. W. (2013). Synergistic childhood adversities and complex adult psychopathology. *Journal of Traumatic Stress, 26*(4), 435–442. https://doi.org/10.1002/jts.21833

Pynoos, R. S., Steinberg, A. M., Layne, C. M., Liang, L.-J., Vivrette, R. L., Briggs, E. C., Kisiel, C., Habib, M., Belin, T. R., & Fairbank, J. A. (2014). Modeling constellations of trauma exposure in the national child traumatic stress network core data set. *Psychological Trauma: Theory, Research, Practice, and Policy, 6*(Suppl 1), S9–S17. https://doi.org/10.1037/a0037767

Pynoos, R. S., Steinberg, A. M., & Piacentini, J. C. (1999). A developmental psychopathology model of childhood traumatic stress and intersection with anxiety disorders. *Biological Psychiatry, 46*(11), 1542–1554. https://doi.org/10.1016/s0006-3223(99)00262-0

Pynoos, R. S., Weathers, F. W., Steinberg, A. M., Marx, B. P., Layne, C. M., Kaloupek, D. G., Schnurr, P. P., Keane, T. M., Blake, D. D., Newman, E., Nafer, K. O., & Kriegler, J. A. (2015). *Clinician-Administered PTSD scale for DSM-5—child/adolescent version.* National Center for PTSD. https://www.ptsd.va.gov/professional/assessment/child/caps-ca.asp

Ribbe, D. (1996). Psychometric review of traumatic events screening inventory for children (TESI-C). In B. Stamm (Ed.), *Measurement of stress, trauma, and adaptation* (pp. 386–387). Sidran Press.

Riediger, M., & Klipker, K. (2014). Emotion regulation in adolescence. In J. J. Gross (Ed.), *Handbook of emotion regulation* (2nd ed., pp. 187–202). Guilford Press.

Riley, F., Bokszczanin, A., & Essau, C. A. (2017). Children of abuse and neglect. In C. A. Essau, S. Leblanc, & T. H. Ollendick (Eds.), *Emotion regulation and psychopathology in children and adolescents* (pp. 305–330). Oxford University Press. https://doi.org/10.1093/med:psych/9780198765844.003.0015

Rizvi, S. L. (2019). *Chain analysis in dialectical behavior therapy.* The Guilford Press.

Sachser, C., Berliner, L., Holt, T., Jensen, T. K., Jungbluth, N., Risch, E., Rosner, R., & Goldbeck, L. (2017). International development and psychometric properties of the child and adolescent trauma screen (CATS). *Journal of Affective Disorders, 210,* 189–195. https://doi.org/10.1016/j.jad.2016.12.040

Saigh, P. A., Yasik, A. E., Oberfield, R. A., Green, B. L., Halamandaris, P. V., Rubenstein, H., Nester, J., Resko, J., Hetz, B., & McHugh, M. (2000). The children's PTSD inventory: Development and reliability. *Journal of Traumatic Stress, 13*(3), 369–380. https://doi.org/10.1023/A:1007750021626

Salloum, A., Stover, C. S., Swaidan, V. R., & Storch, E. A. (2015). Parent and child PTSD and parent depression in relation to parenting stress among trauma-exposed children. *Journal of Child and Family Studies*, *24*(5), 1203–1212. https://doi.org/10.1007/s10826-014-9928-1

Sanjeevi, J., Houlihan, D., Bergstrom, K. A., Langley, M. M., & Judkins, J. (2018). A review of child sexual abuse: Impact, risk, and resilience in the context of culture. *Journal of Child Sexual Abuse*, *27*(6), 622–641. https://doi.org/10.1080/10538712.2018.1486934

Saxe, G., Chawla, N., Stoddard, F., Kassam-Adams, N., Courtney, D., Cunningham, K., Lopez, C., Hall, E., Sheridan, R., King, D., & King, L. (2003). Child stress disorders checklist: A measure of ASD and PTSD in children. *Journal of the American Academy of Child & Adolescent Psychiatry*, *42*(8), 972–978. https://doi.org/10.1097/01.CHI.0000046887.27264.F3

Saxe, G. N., Ellis, B. H., Fogler, J., & Navalta, C. P. (2012). Innovations in practice: Preliminary evidence for effective family engagement in treatment for child traumatic stress–trauma systems therapy approach to preventing dropout. *Child and Adolescent Mental Health*, *17*(1), 58–61. https://doi.org/10.1111/j.1475-3588.2011.00626.x

Saxe, G. N., Ellis, B. H., & Kaplow, J. B. (2007). *Collaborative treatment of traumatized children and teens: The trauma systems therapy approach*. Guilford Press.

Saylor, C. F., Swenson, C. C., Stokes Reynolds, S., & Taylor, M. (1999). The pediatric emotional distress scale: A brief screening measure for young children exposed to traumatic events. *Journal of Clinical Child Psychology*, *28*(1), 70–81. https://doi.org/10.1207/s15374424jccp2801_6

Scheeringa, M. S., & Haslett, N. (2010). The reliability and criterion validity of the diagnostic infant and preschool assessment: A new diagnostic instrument for young children. *Child Psychiatry & Human Development*, *41*(3), 299–312. https://doi.org/10.1007/s10578-009-0169-2

Scheeringa, M. S., & Zeanah, C. H. (2001). A relational perspective on PTSD in early childhood. *Journal of Traumatic Stress*, *14*(4), 799–815. https://doi.org/10.1023/A:1013002507972

Schilpzand, E. J., Conroy, R., Anderson, V., & Alisic, E. (2018). Development and evaluation of the thinking about recovery scale: measure of parent posttraumatic cognitions following children's exposure to trauma. *Journal of Traumatic Stress*, *31*(1), 71–78. https://doi.org/10.1002/jts.22258

Schmid, M., Petermann, F., & Fegert, J. M. (2013). Developmental trauma disorder: Pros and cons of including formal criteria in the psychiatric diagnostic systems. *BMC Psychiatry*, *13*(1), 3. https://doi.org/10.1186/1471-244X-13-3

Schuck, A. M., & Widom, C. S. (2001). Childhood victimization and alcohol symptoms in females: Causal inferences and hypothesized mediators. *Child Abuse & Neglect*, *25*(8), 1069–1092. https://doi.org/10.1016/S0145-2134(01)00257-5

Sedlak, A. J., Mettenburg, J., Basena, M., Petta, I., McPherson, K., Greene, A., & Li, S. (2010). *Fourth national incidence study of child abuse and neglect (NIS–4): Report to congress, executive summary.* U.S. Department of Health and Human Services, Administration for Children and Families. https://www.acf.hhs.gov/sites/default/files/documents/opre/nis4_report_exec_summ_pdf_jan2010.pdf

Shackman, J. E., Shackman, A. J., & Pollak, S. D. (2007). Physical abuse amplifies attention to threat and increases anxiety in children. *Emotion, 7*(4), 838–852. https://doi.org/10.1037/1528-3542.7.4.838

Shaffer, A., Kotchick, B. A., Dorsey, S., & Forehand, R. (2001). The past, present, and future of behavioral parent training: Interventions for child and adolescent problem behavior. *The Behavior Analyst Today, 2*(2), 91–105. https://doi.org/10.1037/h0099922

Shields, A., & Cicchetti, D. (1997). Emotion regulation among school-age children: The development and validation of a new criterion Q-sort scale. *Developmental Psychology, 33*(6), 906–916. https://doi.org/10.1037/0012-1649.33.6.906

Shochet, I., & Dadds, M. (1997). When individual child psychotherapy exacerbates family systems problems in child abuse cases: A clinical analysis. *Clinical Child Psychology and Psychiatry, 2*(2), 239–249. https://doi.org/10.1177/1359104597022005

Silverman, W. K., & Albano, A. M. (1996). *Anxiety disorders interview schedule for DSM-IV.* Oxford University Press.

Simmons, D. (2008). Epigenetic influence and disease. *Nature Education, 1*(1), 6. https://www.nature.com/scitable/topicpage/epigenetic-influences-and-disease-895/

Skowron, E. A., Cipriano-Essel, E., Gatzke-Kopp, L. M., Teti, D. M., & Ammerman, R. T. (2014). Early adversity, RSA, and inhibitory control: Evidence of children's neurobiological sensitivity to social context. *Developmental Psychobiology, 56*(5), 964–978. https://doi.org/10.1002/dev.21175

Smith, P. (Ed.) (2010). *Post traumatic stress disorder: Cognitive therapy with children and young people.* Routledge.

Sointu, E. T., Savolainen, H., Lambert, M. C., Lappalainen, K., & Epstein, M. H. (2014). Behavioral and emotional strength-based assessment of Finnish elementary students: Psychometrics of the BERS-2. *European Journal of Psychology of Education, 29*(1), 1–19. psyh. https://doi.org/10.1007/s10212-013-0184-3

Southwick, S. M., Bonanno, G. A., Masten, A. S., Panter-Brick, C., & Yehuda, R. (2014). Resilience definitions, theory, and challenges: Interdisciplinary perspectives. *European Journal of Psychotraumatology, 5*(1), 25338. https://doi.org/10.3402/ejpt.v5.25338

Spinazzola, J., Ford, J. D., Zucker, M., van der Kolk, B. A., Silva, S., Smith, S. F., & Blaustein, M. (2005). National survey of complex trauma exposure, outcome and intervention for children and adolescents. *Psychiatric Annals, 35*(5), 433–439. https://doi.org/10.3928/00485713-20050501-09

Sroufe, L. A., & Rutter, M. (1984). The domain of developmental psychopathology. *Child Development, 55*(1), 17–29.

Stallard, P. (2003). A retrospective analysis to explore the applicability of the Ehlers and Clark (2000) cognitive model to explain PTSD in children. *Behavioural and Cognitive Psychotherapy, 31*(3), 337–345. https://doi.org/10 .1017/S1352465803003084

Stegge, H., & Terwogt, M. M. (2007). Awareness and regulation of emotion in typical and atypical development. In J. J. Gross (Ed.), *Handbook of emotion regulation.* (pp. 269–286). Guilford Press.

Stensland, S. O., Thoresen, S., Wentzel-Larsen, T., Zwart, J.-A., & Dyb, G. (2014). Recurrent headache and interpersonal violence in adolescence: The roles of psychological distress, loneliness and family cohesion: the HUNT study. *The Journal of Headache and Pain, 15*, 35. https://doi.org/10.1186/1129-2377-15-35

Stoddard, J., Reynolds, E. K., Paris, R., Haller, S., Johnson, S., Zik, J., Elliote, E., Maru, M., Jaffe, A., Mallidi, A., Smith, A., Hernandez, R. G., Volk, H. E., Brotman, M. A., & Kaufman, J. (2021). *The coronavirus impact scale: construction, validation, and comparisons in diverse clinical samples* [Preprint]. PsyArXiv. https://doi.org/10.31234/osf.io/kz4pg

Stolbach, B. C., Minshew, R., Rompala, V., Dominguez, R. Z., Gazibara, T., & Finke, R. (2013). Complex trauma exposure and symptoms in urban traumatized children: A preliminary test of proposed criteria for developmental trauma disorder: Complex trauma in the lives of urban children. *Journal of Traumatic Stress, 26*(4), 483–491. https://doi.org/10.1002/jts.21826

Sue, D. W., Capodilupo, C. M., Torino, G. C., Bucceri, J. M., Holder, A. M. B., Nadal, K. L., & Esquilin, M. (2007). Racial microaggressions in everyday life: Implications for clinical practice. *The American Psychologist, 62*(4), 271–286. https://doi.org/10.1037/0003-066X.62.4.271

Symes, L., McFarlane, J., Fredland, N., Maddoux, J., & Zhou, W. (2016). Parenting in the wake of abuse: Exploring the mediating role of PTSD symptoms on the relationship between parenting and child functioning. *Archives of Psychiatric Nursing, 30*(1), 90–95. https://doi.org/10.1016/j.apnu.2015.08.020

Teicher, M. H., & Samson, J. A. (2016). Annual research review: Enduring neurobiological effects of childhood abuse and neglect. *Journal of Child Psychology and Psychiatry, 57*(3), 241–266. https://doi.org/10.1111/jcpp.12507

Teicher, M. H., Samson, J. A., Polcari, A., & McGreenery, C. E. (2006). Sticks, stones, and hurtful words: Relative effects of various forms of childhood maltreatment. *American Journal of Psychiatry, 163*(6), 993–1000. https://doi .org/10.1176/ajp.2006.163.6.993

Terr, L. C. (1979). Children of chowchilla: A study of psychic trauma. *The Psychoanalytic Study of the Child, 34*(1), 547–623. https://doi.org/10.1080/ 00797308.1979.11823018

Thompson, R. A. (1994). Emotion regulation: A theme in search of definition. *Monographs of the Society for Research in Child Development*, *59*(2–3), 25–52. https://doi.org/10.2307/1166137

Thompson, R. A. (2019). Emotion dysregulation: A theme in search of definition. *Development and Psychopathology*, *31*(3), 805–815. https://doi.org/10.1017/S0954579419000282

Thompson, R. A., & Goodman, M. (2010). Development of emotion regulation: More than meets the eye. In A. M. Kring & D. M. Sloan (Eds.), *Emotion regulation and psychopathology: A transdiagnostic approach to etiology and treatment*. (pp. 38–58). Guilford Press.

Tomoda, A., Sheu, Y.-S., Rabi, K., Suzuki, H., Navalta, C. P., Polcari, A., & Teicher, M. H. (2011). Exposure to parental verbal abuse is associated with increased gray matter volume in superior temporal gyrus. *NeuroImage*, *54*, S280–S286. https://doi.org/10.1016/j.neuroimage.2010.05.027

Trent, M., Dooley, D. G., & Dougé, J. SECTION ON ADOLESCENT HEALTH, COUNCIL ON COMMUNITY PEDIATRICS, & COMMITTEE ON ADOLESCENCE (2019). The impact of racism on child and adolescent health. *Pediatrics*, *144*(2), e20191765. https://doi.org/10.1542/peds.2019-1765

Trickey, D., Siddaway, A. P., Meiser-Stedman, R., Serpell, L., & Field, A. P. (2012). A meta-analysis of risk factors for post-traumatic stress disorder in children and adolescents. *Clinical Psychology Review*, *32*(2), 122–138. https://doi.org/10.1016/j.cpr.2011.12.001

Trimble, M. (1981). *Post-traumatic neurosis: From railway spine to the whiplash*. John Wiley & Sons Ltd.

Trocme, N., & Caunce, C. (1995). The educational needs of abused and neglected children: A review of the literature. *Early Child Development and Care*, *106*(1), 101–135. https://doi.org/10.1080/0300443951060110

Truscott, D. (2010). *Becoming an effective psychotherapist: Adopting a theory of psychotherapy that's right for you and your client*. American Psychological Association. https://doi.org/10.1037/12064-000

U.S. Census Bureau. (2021). *2020 census state redistricting data (public law 94-171) summary file*. https://www2.census.gov/programs-surveys/decennial/2020/technical-documentation/complete-tech-docs/summary-file/2020Census_PL94_171Redistricting_StatesTechDoc_English.pdf#page=160

U.S. Department of Health & Human Services, Administration for Children and Families, & Administration on Children, Youth and Families, Children's Bureau. (2020). *Child maltreatment 2018*. https://www.acf.hhs.gov/cb/data-research/child-maltreatment

van Der Kolk, B., Ford, J. D., & Spinazzola, J. (2019). Comorbidity of developmental trauma disorder (DTD) and post-traumatic stress disorder: Findings from the DTD field trial. *European Journal of Psychotraumatology*, *10*(1), 1562841. https://doi.org/10.1080/20008198.2018.1562841

van Der Kolk, B., Pynoos, R. S., Cicchetti, D., Cloitre, M., D'Andrea, W., Ford, J. D., & Teicher, M. H. (2009). *Proposal to include a developmental trauma disorder diagnosis for children and adolescents in DSM-V*.

Veltman, M. W. M., & Browne, K. D. (2001). Three decades of child maltreatment research: Implications for the school years. *Trauma, Violence, & Abuse, 2*(3), 215–239. https://doi.org/10.1177/1524838001002003002

Vissing, Y. M., Straus, M. A., Gelles, R. J., & Harrop, J. W. (1991). Verbal aggression by parents and psychosocial problems of children. *Child Abuse & Neglect, 15*(3), 223–238. https://doi.org/10.1016/0145-2134(91)90067-N

Waldrop, A. E., Hanson, R. F., Resnick, H. S., Kilpatrick, D. G., Naugle, A. E., & Saunders, B. E. (2007). Risk factors for suicidal behavior among a national sample of adolescents: Implications for prevention. *Journal of Traumatic Stress, 20*(5), 869–879. https://doi.org/10.1002/jts.20291

Weisaeth, L. (1984). *Stress reactions to an industrial disaster*. Medical Faculty, University of Oslo.

Werner, K., & Gross, J. J. (2010). Emotion regulation and psychopathology: A conceptual framework. In A. M. Kring & D. M. Sloan (Eds.), *Emotion regulation and psychopathology: A transdiagnostic approach to etiology and treatment.* (pp. 13–37). Guilford Press.

Whitfield, C. L., Dube, S. R., Felitti, V. J., & Anda, R. F. (2005). Adverse childhood experiences and hallucinations. *Child Abuse & Neglect, 29*(7), 797–810. https://doi.org/10.1016/j.chiabu.2005.01.004

Wilens, T. E., & Hammerness, P. G. (2016). *Straight talk about psychiatric medications for kids* (4th ed.). The Guilford Press.

Williams, M. T., Metzger, I. W., Leins, C., & DeLapp, C. (2018). Assessing racial trauma within a DSM–5 framework: The UConn Racial/Ethnic Stress & Trauma Survey. *Practice Innovations, 3*(4), 242–260. https://doi.org/10.1037/pri0000076

Williamson, V., Hiller, R. M., Meiser-Stedman, R., Creswell, C., Dalgleish, T., Fearon, P., Goodall, B., McKinnon, A., Smith, P., Wright, I., & Halligan, S. L. (2018). The parent trauma response questionnaire (PTRQ): Development and preliminary validation. *European Journal of Psychotraumatology, 9*(1), 1478583. https://doi.org/10.1080/20008198.2018.1478583

Winters, N. C., Hanson, G., & Stoyanova, V. (2007). The case formulation in child and adolescent psychiatry. *Child and Adolescent Psychiatric Clinics of North America, 16*(1), 111–132. https://doi.org/10.1016/j.chc.2006.07.010

Wodarski, J. S., Kurtz, P. D., Gaudin, J. M., & Howing, P. T. (1990). Maltreatment and the school-age child: Major academic, socioemotional, and adaptive outcomes. *Social Work, 35*(6), 506–513. https://doi.org/10.1093/sw/35.6.506

Woo, B. (2018). Racial discrimination and mental health in the USA: Testing the reverse racism hypothesis. *Journal of Racial and Ethnic Health Disparities, 5*(4), 766–773. https://doi.org/10.1007/s40615-017-0421-6

World Health Organization. (2001). *International classification of functioning, disability and health (ICF)*.

World Health Organization. (2018). *International classification of diseases 11th revision (ICD-11)*. WHO. https://icd.who.int/en

World Health Organization, Regional Office for South-East Asia. (2009). *Self-care in the context of primary health care*. WHO Regional Office for South-East Asia. https://apps.who.int/iris/handle/10665/206352

Zimmer-Gembeck, M. J., & Skinner, E. A. (2016). The development of coping: Implications for psychopathology and resilience. In D. Cicchetti (Ed.), *Developmental psychopathology* (pp. 1–61). John Wiley & Sons, Inc. https://doi.org/10.1002/9781119125556.devpsy410

Index

Page numbers in *italics* denote figures and numbers in **bold** denote tables.

Trauma-Informed Parenting Program: TIPˢ for Clinicians to Train Parents of Children Impacted by Trauma & Adversity, First Edition. Carryl P. Navalta.
© 2022 John Wiley & Sons, Inc. Published 2022 by John Wiley & Sons, Inc.
Companion Website: www.wiley.com/go/navalta/tipsforclinicians

Printed and bound by CPI Group (UK) Ltd, Croydon, CR0 4YY

10/03/2024

14467727-0001